REVERSING DIABETES
10 Natural Secrets to Reverse Diabetes Without Drugs

Dr. Joseph Jacobs, DPT, ACN

First Edition, January 2026
Published by ASTR Institute
614 E HWY 50 #169, Clermont, FL 34711

ASTR

ASTRinstitute.com

The author and publisher have made every effort to ensure the accuracy of the information herein, but the information contained in this book is sold without warranty, either express or implied. Neither the author nor the publisher will be held liable for any damages caused, directly or indirectly, by the instructions contained in this book.

Disclaimer

This book, authored by Dr. Joseph Jacobs and published by the ASTR Institute, is intended for informational purposes only and presents medical research findings. It is not a substitute for professional medical advice, diagnosis, or treatment. Dr. Joseph Jacobs, the ASTR Institute, and its affiliates do not endorse or assume responsibility for any specific medical treatments or procedures discussed in this book. We strongly advise readers to consult with their healthcare providers regarding the applicability of any aspects of the content to their own health and well-being.

The statements contained herein have not been evaluated by the Food and Drug Administration. The products mentioned are not designed to diagnose, cure, treat, or prevent any disease. Individual results may vary, and we cannot guarantee that you will achieve the same outcomes as those detailed in our case studies, testimonials, and treatment videos. Success varies per individual, and one person's results do not guarantee similar outcomes for another.

If you have medical concerns, consult with your healthcare provider, physician, or another qualified medical professional. Dr. Joseph Jacobs, the ASTR Institute, and their associated organizations and individuals disclaim any liability for actions, services, or products acquired through this book, our videos, website, or any of our media channels.

Table of Contents

Online Resources

How to Access Online Resources

Throughout this book, you'll find barcodes that link to additional online resources. Here's how to use them:

1. Open the camera app on your smartphone.
2. Point the camera at the barcode.
3. A notification will appear with a link. Tap the notification to open the link in your browser.

Triumph Over Trials: My Journey from Disability to Victory

After my second cancer treatment, I was suffering from chronic fatigue, migraines, muscle and joint pain. I reached out to at least seven doctors, but I could not find relief. Unfortunately, they had two responses. First, they said my blood labs looked normal. I learned from my studies in nutrition that this happened because they did not order the correct labs to figure out the root cause of my issues. The second response was that I was a hopeless case. This made me realize that if I wanted to overcome my disability, I had to look for a solution on my own. It was a difficult time in my life. Due to my pain and fatigue, it used to take me 10 minutes just to walk from the living room to the bathroom, about 20 feet away. I was very depressed and angry because, at 30 years old, I was facing numerous health issues and had a poor quality of life without any answers.

I spent countless hours and years studying nutrition, psychology, behavioral modification, anatomy, physiology, ergonomics, and other medical topics in hopes of finding an answer. At the same time, I was frustrated that the techniques I learned in medical school only provided short-term results with no lasting relief. I tried what I learned in school, such as stretching, exercises, electrical stimulation, various massage techniques, manual therapy, joint mobilization, and myofascial release, but nothing provided long-term results. So, I started to look at medical studies to guide me through this process. After reviewing over 16,000 medical research papers with assistance from medical students, I was shocked and disappointed by the results. Based on these studies, the following treatments either provided no pain reduction or only short-term pain reduction:

- NSAIDs
- Opioids
- Cortisone shots
- Exercises
- Stretching
- Massage
- Joint mobilization or manipulation
- Acupuncture
- Dry needling
- Instrument-assisted soft tissue mobilization

I have dedicated my life to researching all current traditional medical approaches to treating pain. I've found that the majority of these approaches primarily focus on relieving symptoms rather than addressing the root cause of the pain. The techniques I learned in school, still used in today's modern medical world, have their origins in ancient healing practices such as manipulation, massage, stretching, and exercise. These methods were used by the Romans, Greeks, and Egyptians to increase flexibility, strengthen muscles, and alleviate pain. Today's medicine has added treatments like cold, heat, electrical stimulation, and joint adjustment to this list. However, overwhelming evidence from published medical studies shows no promising long-term relief from any of these methods.

For instance, one systematic review conducted by the University of Ottawa, Canada, which reviewed 270 research studies, concluded that the benefits of massage, acupuncture, and spine adjustment treatments were mostly evident immediately or shortly after treatment, then faded over time. With compelling data like this, it is perplexing how we continue to treat patients with modalities that do not effectively address their long-term needs. Instead of focusing so much on the body's symptoms, we need to start questioning why these symptoms are present in the first place and why they keep returning.

This question guided me through an intense investigative research process over five years. From this research, I concluded that there are seven aspects of chronic pain that, when treated simultaneously, can lead to long-term pain relief. In my book, **Pain No More**, I outline seven key elements that must be addressed simultaneously to effectively relieve chronic pain. I also found that the BioPsychosocial model is an effective treatment approach for long-term pain reduction. So, I studied the BioPsychosocial model in depth and realized that my medical education was lacking in nutrition knowledge. I spent thousands of hours reading and studying nutrition and bought any book that I felt could help me understand the body better.

During this time, my wife had chronic jaw pain due to stress at work. I tried everything I learned from school on her, but nothing provided long-term pain relief. One day she woke up with lockjaw, unable to speak or open her mouth. She asked me to try anything. I told her that I had tried everything I knew, but nothing worked. So, I reached inside her mouth and experimented with several maneuvers. After a few minutes, she was able to open her mouth and was pain-free. I was dumbfounded and had no idea what had just happened. It took me several days to understand the physiology of the maneuvers I had performed. I then started experimenting with the same concept, applying it to the whole body to relieve both my pain and my patients' pain.

After several months of using my hands to implement the new maneuvers I had come up with, I realized I could not do that long-term. My hands were very sore, and I suffered from pain every night. I told my wife that this was not sustainable because I was in so much pain from using my hands. While patients were getting relief, I was suffering. My wife suggested that I use tools instead of my hands. So, I went to a hardware store and bought rubber, plastic, and metal to cut and design tools and devices to replace my hand maneuvers. Thankfully, this provided even faster results for my patients without me feeling soreness from working on them.

I was able to overcome my chronic fatigue and migraines by running comprehensive lab tests. These tests revealed several vitamin, mineral, and hormonal imbalances. Additionally, I overcame my chronic joint and muscle pain through the biopsychosocial (BPS) model and the tools and devices I invented. I also reinvented the biopsychosocial model to be implemented by a single healthcare provider and called it ASTR treatment.

My journey toward developing the ASTR diet was driven by personal challenges and professional insights. I experienced significant frustration with various diets that often left me feeling fatigued and unsatisfied. Through an extensive review of research studies, I also uncovered potential health risks associated with extreme dietary approaches. These experiences inspired me to create the ASTR Diet as a healthier, evidence-based alternative, which I share in my book **Eat to Heal**.

For years, I suffered from debilitating migraines, searching for lasting relief beyond temporary fixes. My journey as both a patient and a healthcare provider led me to dedicate 15 years to researching, studying, and testing effective solutions. Through this process, I developed a comprehensive approach that transformed my own health and has helped countless patients overcome chronic pain and chronic disease.. In this book, I share these evidence-based strategies, solutions that I have refined through experience and clinical practice. My hope is that this book serves as a practical guide to empower you on your path to recovery, providing the tools and knowledge you need to reclaim your health and live diabetes free.

Understanding Diabetes

Diabetes mellitus is a chronic metabolic disorder characterized by elevated blood glucose levels due to insufficient insulin production, impaired insulin action, or both. Understanding the underlying physiology, risk factors, and diagnostic markers of diabetes is essential for effective prevention and management.

Pancreatic Function

The pancreas is central to glucose regulation. It contains clusters of cells known as the islets of Langerhans, where beta cells produce insulin and alpha cells produce glucagon. Insulin promotes glucose uptake into muscle and adipose tissues, while glucagon increases blood glucose during fasting (Röder et al., 2016). Damage to pancreatic beta cells leads to insulin deficiency, contributing to the development of diabetes.

The pancreas and liver work together to regulate blood sugar, but they serve very different roles. The pancreas produces hormones, not glucose storage. Its beta cells release insulin, which helps move glucose into cells for energy or storage, while its alpha cells release glucagon, which signals the liver during fasting or low blood sugar. The liver is the primary storage site for glycogen, the stored form of glucose. When blood sugar drops, glucagon tells the liver to break down glycogen into glucose and release it into the bloodstream, helping maintain stable blood sugar levels between meals and during periods without food.

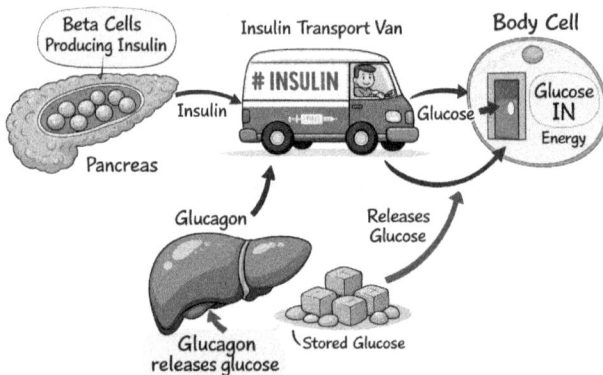

Liver Function

The liver maintains glucose homeostasis through glycogenolysis (breakdown of glycogen to glucose) and gluconeogenesis (production of glucose from non-carbohydrate sources). In individuals with type 2 diabetes, insulin resistance often results in uncontrolled hepatic glucose production, contributing significantly to hyperglycemia (Rui, 2014).

Types of Diabetes

Diabetes is broadly classified into two main types:
Type 1 Diabetes (T1D): An autoimmune condition in which the immune system destroys pancreatic beta cells. It typically presents in childhood or adolescence and requires lifelong insulin therapy (American Diabetes Association [ADA], 2023). **Type 2 Diabetes (T2D):** Characterized by insulin resistance and relative insulin deficiency. It is associated with poor dietary habits, obesity, and physical inactivity and represents the majority of diabetes cases (ADA, 2023).

Symptoms of Diabetes

The clinical presentation of diabetes varies by type:

Type 1 Diabetes Symptoms
Common symptoms of type 1 diabetes include:
- Polyuria, frequent urination
- Polydipsia, increased thirst
- Polyphagia, increased hunger
- Unexplained weight loss
- Fatigue and irritability
- Blurred vision

Type 2 Diabetes Symptoms
Common symptoms of type 2 diabetes include:
- Fatigue
- Frequent infections
- Slow-healing wounds

- Blurred vision
- Tingling or numbness in the hands or feet
- Unexplained weight changes

Prediabetes

Prediabetes is a health condition in which blood sugar levels are higher than normal but not yet high enough to be diagnosed as type 2 diabetes. It serves as a critical warning sign, indicating that the body is beginning to lose its ability to manage blood glucose effectively. This condition typically develops when the body's cells become resistant to insulin or when the pancreas cannot produce enough insulin to maintain normal glucose levels. According to the Centers for Disease Control and Prevention (CDC), more than 1 in 3 American adults has prediabetes, yet over 80% of them are unaware of their condition.

Prediabetes is closely associated with **metabolic syndrome**, a cluster of risk factors including abdominal obesity, elevated triglycerides, low HDL cholesterol, high blood pressure, and elevated fasting glucose. These metabolic disturbances not only increase the risk of developing type 2 diabetes but also significantly raise the risk of cardiovascular disease. The underlying causes of prediabetes often include a combination of genetic predisposition, poor dietary habits, sedentary lifestyle, chronic stress, sleep disturbances, and exposure to environmental toxins.

Lab indicators used to diagnose prediabetes include a fasting blood glucose level between 100–125 mg/dL, an HbA1c level between 5.6%–6.4%, or a 2-hour oral glucose tolerance test (OGTT) result between 140–199 mg/dL. These markers reflect early glucose dysregulation and are used to initiate early interventions aimed at preventing progression to diabetes. Studies show that lifestyle interventions such as improving diet quality, increasing physical activity, reducing body weight, and managing stress can cut the risk of developing type 2 diabetes by more than 50% (Knowler et al., 2002).

Prediabetes is often silent, with no obvious symptoms, which is why routine screening is crucial, especially for individuals who are overweight, have a family history of diabetes, or are over the age of 45. When symptoms do appear, they may include increased thirst, frequent urination, fatigue, or blurred vision, although these are more common in later stages. Early detection and intervention are essential, as reversing prediabetes is possible with sustained lifestyle changes. Without such changes, most individuals with prediabetes will develop type 2 diabetes within five to ten years.

Metabolic Syndrome and Diabetes

Metabolic syndrome is a cluster of interrelated conditions including central obesity, hypertension, elevated triglycerides, low HDL cholesterol, and insulin resistance that significantly increases the risk of developing type 2 diabetes and cardiovascular disease. Individuals with metabolic syndrome often experience chronic low-grade inflammation and hormonal imbalances that disrupt normal glucose metabolism. According to the National Heart, Lung, and Blood Institute, having three or more of these risk factors qualifies as a diagnosis of metabolic syndrome, which affects an estimated one-third of U.S. adults (Grundy et al., 2005).

The link between metabolic syndrome and diabetes lies in insulin resistance, a condition in which the body's cells become less responsive to insulin. This leads to higher blood sugar levels. Over time, the pancreas struggles to keep up with the increased demand for insulin, eventually leading to beta-cell dysfunction and the onset of type 2 diabetes. This progression is often accelerated by poor diet, physical inactivity, and excess abdominal fat. These are all factors that directly contribute to metabolic syndrome.

Moreover, metabolic syndrome not only increases the likelihood of developing type 2 diabetes but also worsens outcomes for those already diagnosed. Individuals with both conditions have a significantly higher risk of complications such as heart disease, kidney dysfunction, and non-alcoholic fatty liver disease (NAFLD). Addressing the root causes of metabolic syndrome through lifestyle interventions such as dietary changes, weight loss, regular exercise, and stress reduction can dramatically lower the risk of diabetes and improve metabolic health.

Hypothalamic-Pituitary-Adrenal (HPA) Axis

The hypothalamic-pituitary-adrenal (HPA) axis is a central neuroendocrine system that regulates the body's response to stress. It functions through a cascade of hormonal signals beginning in the hypothalamus, which stimulates the pituitary gland to release adrenocorticotropic hormone (ACTH). ACTH then prompts the adrenal glands to secrete cortisol, the primary stress hormone. While this system is vital for adapting to acute stress, chronic activation of the HPA axis can have detrimental metabolic effects.

In individuals with or at risk for diabetes, chronic stress and sustained HPA axis activation contribute to elevated cortisol levels, which in turn impair insulin sensitivity and promote gluconeogenesis, leading to persistent hyperglycemia. Elevated cortisol also favors the accumulation of visceral fat, which further exacerbates insulin resistance. Over time, this hormonal dysregulation can contribute to the development and progression of type 2 diabetes.

The HPA Axis, Stress, and Diabetes

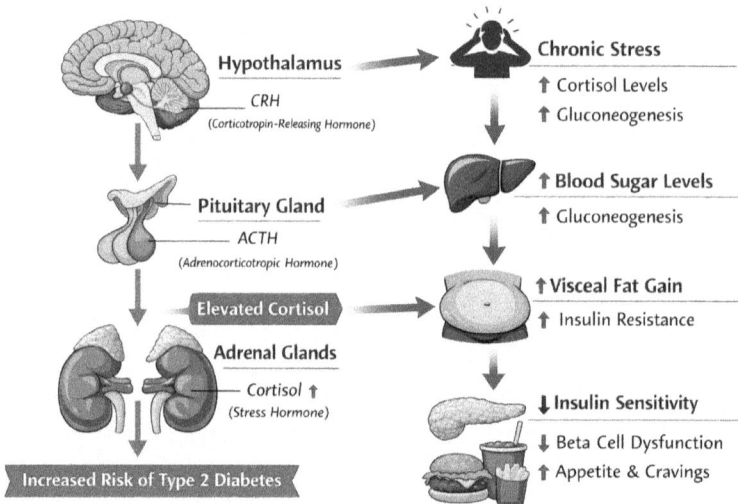

Hypothalamus

CRH
(Corticotropin-Releasing Hormone)

Pituitary Gland

ACTH
(Adrenocorticotropic Hormone)

Elevated Cortisol

Adrenal Glands

Cortisol ↑
(Stress Hormone)

Increased Risk of Type 2 Diabetes

Chronic Stress
↑ Cortisol Levels
↑ Gluconeogenesis

↑ Blood Sugar Levels
↑ Gluconeogenesis

↑ Visceal Fat Gain
↑ Insulin Resistance

↓ Insulin Sensitivity
↓ Beta Cell Dysfunction
↑ Appetite & Cravings

Furthermore, elevated cortisol levels can disrupt pancreatic beta-cell function and increase appetite, particularly cravings for high-sugar and high-fat foods, contributing to weight gain and metabolic syndrome. These effects underscore the importance of stress management in the prevention and management of diabetes.

Risk Factors

Key risk factors for developing diabetes include:

- Family history of diabetes
- Obesity or being overweight
- Sedentary lifestyle
- High carbohydrate intake
- Advanced age
- Certain ethnic backgrounds, including African American, Hispanic, Native American, and Asian American
- Polycystic ovary syndrome
- History of gestational diabetes

Physiology of Diabetes

Insulin facilitates the transport of glucose from the bloodstream into cells. In type 2 diabetes, insulin resistance diminishes this process, leading to elevated blood glucose levels. Prolonged hyperglycemia contributes to vascular and nerve damage, increasing the risk for neuropathy, nephropathy, retinopathy, and cardiovascular complications (DeFronzo et al., 2015).

The diagnosis of diabetes is based on specific laboratory values:

- Fasting Plasma Glucose (FPG): ≥126 mg/dL (7.0 mmol/L)
- 2-Hour Oral Glucose Tolerance Test (OGTT): ≥200 mg/dL (11.1 mmol/L)
- Hemoglobin A1C (HbA1c): ≥6.5%, reflecting average blood glucose levels over the past two to three months (ADA, 2023)

In addition to these diagnostic criteria, fasting insulin levels are a valuable early detection marker for insulin resistance, which often develops years before fasting glucose or A1C levels become abnormal. Elevated fasting insulin can signal metabolic dysfunction at an earlier stage, allowing for earlier intervention and prevention of progression to type 2 diabetes.

Diabetes Statistics

According to the CDC (2023), an estimated 37.3 million Americans live with diabetes, and nearly 96 million have prediabetes. Alarmingly, one in five individuals with diabetes is unaware of their condition. Diabetes ranks as the seventh leading cause of death in the United States.

Diabetes Complications

Chronic hyperglycemia damages both small and large blood vessels, leading to a range of complications that affect nearly every organ system.

- **Diabetic Neuropathy:** Nerve damage that often begins in the feet, leading to pain, numbness, tingling, balance problems, ulcers, and in severe cases, limb loss.
- **Diabetic Nephropathy:** Progressive kidney damage that impairs filtration and is a leading cause of chronic kidney disease and end-stage renal failure.
- **Diabetic Retinopathy:** Damage to the small blood vessels of the retina, increasing the risk of vision loss and blindness.
- **Coronary Artery Disease:** Increased risk of heart attacks due to accelerated atherosclerosis and vascular inflammation.
- **Stroke:** Higher likelihood of ischemic and hemorrhagic stroke as a result of vascular damage and impaired blood flow regulation.
- **Peripheral Arterial Disease:** Reduced blood flow to the limbs, contributing to pain, poor wound healing, infections, and amputations.
- **Impaired Immune Function:** Increased susceptibility to infections and delayed recovery due to chronic hyperglycemia.
- **Delayed Wound Healing:** Poor circulation and nerve damage increase the risk of chronic wounds, ulcers, and secondary infections.

Conclusion

Diabetes is a complex, multifactorial condition shaped by genetic, hormonal, environmental, and behavioral influences. This book is specifically written for individuals with **prediabetes and type 2 diabetes**, where prevention, stabilization, and reversal are most achievable. In these stages, metabolic dysfunction is largely driven by insulin resistance, nutrient and hormonal imbalances, chronic stress, poor sleep, and lifestyle-related exposures rather than irreversible pancreatic failure.

Effective prevention and treatment require addressing these root causes, not simply managing blood sugar levels. By focusing on dietary changes, consistent physical activity, stress regulation, sleep optimization, toxin reduction, and targeted nutritional support, the body can restore metabolic balance and improve insulin sensitivity. When these factors are addressed together, individuals with prediabetes and type 2 diabetes can significantly reduce disease progression, improve blood sugar control, and reclaim long-term metabolic health.

Case Studies and Research

Research Supporting the 10 Natural Secrets

<u>Case Study 1:</u> From 500 to 89: Restoring Blood Sugar Control Through Natural Metabolic Healing

This case demonstrates how addressing the root causes of insulin resistance through a structured, natural approach can lead to profound improvements in blood sugar control when implemented consistently and under appropriate medical supervision. A middle-aged female patient presented to the emergency room with **critically elevated blood glucose levels exceeding 500 mg/dL**. At this level, blood sugar is dangerously high and places severe strain on the pancreas, kidneys, cardiovascular system, and nervous system. Like many individuals with underlying insulin resistance, her condition had developed gradually and largely unnoticed over time. She reported experiencing warning signs including persistent fatigue, excessive thirst, frequent urination, brain fog, and unstable energy levels. These symptoms were present for months, yet they were not initially recognized as indicators of progressing metabolic dysfunction.

The patient made a conscious decision to address the **root causes** of her elevated blood sugar rather than relying solely on crisis-based care. With appropriate medical oversight, she began implementing the principles outlined in this book, focusing on the Ten Natural Secrets for Reversing Insulin Resistance and Restoring Metabolic Health.

Her approach included targeted dietary changes using an anti-inflammatory, toxin-free nutritional strategy, elimination of blood sugar triggers, improved hydration and mineral balance, structured meal timing, stress reduction, gentle daily movement, and behavioral changes designed to support long-term metabolic stability. Her plan also included individualized vitamin and mineral support based on documented deficiencies identified through blood work. Each component was implemented intentionally, recognizing that diabetes is a complex condition requiring a comprehensive and integrated strategy.

The patient experienced a steady and measurable improvement in her blood sugar levels. Through consistency and adherence to the full framework, her fasting and daily glucose readings normalized. Ultimately, her blood sugar decreased from **over 500 mg/dL to 89 mg/dL**, placing her well within a healthy range.

Equally important, her symptoms improved significantly. She reported increased energy, clearer thinking and a renewed sense of control over her health. This transformation highlights what is possible when insulin resistance is addressed early and holistically, rather than managed reactively. This case underscores a critical message of this book: diabetes does not begin in the emergency room, and healing does not end with a prescription. When the underlying drivers of insulin resistance are identified and corrected, the body has a remarkable capacity to restore balance.

To watch the patient's video interview discussing her case and results, scan the QR code.

Case Study 2: **From the 300s on Insulin to Stable Control: Improving Blood Sugar Through Integrated Lifestyle Intervention**

This case highlights how implementing a comprehensive, root-cause–based approach can significantly improve blood sugar control, even in individuals with long-standing diabetes requiring multiple medications and insulin therapy. My father had a history of poorly controlled blood sugar, with **glucose levels frequently ranging in the 300 mg/dL range**. During a prior hospitalization, his blood sugar remained elevated despite receiving **insulin therapy under medical supervision**. While hospitalized, he consumed standard hospital meals, which are often high in refined carbohydrates and processed ingredients, making glucose control difficult even with aggressive pharmacologic intervention. At the time of discharge and in the weeks that followed, my father was prescribed **six separate dosages of blood sugar medications daily**, yet his glucose readings continued to fluctuate between **200 and 300 mg/dL**. Despite adherence to his medication regimen, his blood sugar remained unstable, reflecting the reality that medications alone often do not address the underlying drivers of insulin resistance.

When my father came to visit me in Florida for one week, we decided to take a different approach. With full awareness of his medical history and while continuing his prescribed medications, we implemented the Ten Natural Secrets outlined in this book, focusing on correcting the metabolic, nutritional, behavioral, and lifestyle factors contributing to his blood sugar dysregulation. Based on his laboratory results, I also provided targeted vitamin and mineral support to address deficiencies.

During this week, we prioritized whole, anti-inflammatory foods, removed refined carbohydrates and blood sugar triggers, optimized hydration and mineral intake, structured meal timing, incorporated gentle daily movement, emphasized restorative sleep, reduced environmental stressors, and addressed behavioral patterns that influence metabolic stability. Each step was implemented intentionally, recognizing that diabetes is a complex condition requiring a coordinated, systems-based strategy.

The results were both rapid and measurable. Within days, my father's blood sugar readings **stabilized between 108 and 124 mg/dL**, a dramatic improvement from his prior range. Importantly, this improvement occurred while his medication burden was reduced from **six daily dosages to just two**, under appropriate oversight. He reported feeling more energetic, mentally clearer, and more confident in his ability to manage his condition.

This case demonstrates a critical principle emphasized throughout this book: medications can support blood sugar control, but they cannot compensate for metabolic dysfunction driven by diet, lifestyle, stress, and environmental factors. When these root causes are addressed together, insulin sensitivity can improve significantly, allowing for better glucose regulation and, in some cases, reduced reliance on medication. While this experience reflects an individual case and outcomes will vary, it reinforces the importance of implementing all ten natural strategies together rather than in isolation. Diabetes management is not about

The Biopsychosocial Model Explained

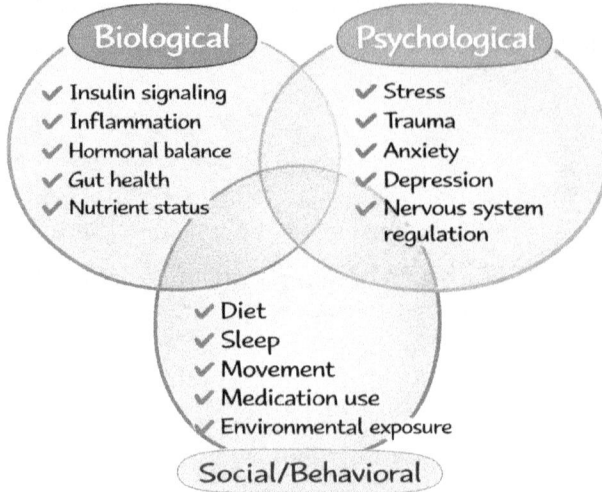

Biological
- ✔ Insulin signaling
- ✔ Inflammation
- ✔ Hormonal balance
- ✔ Gut health
- ✔ Nutrient status

Psychological
- ✔ Stress
- ✔ Trauma
- ✔ Anxiety
- ✔ Depression
- ✔ Nervous system regulation

- ✔ Diet
- ✔ Sleep
- ✔ Movement
- ✔ Medication use
- ✔ Environmental exposure

Social/Behavioral

willpower or restriction; it is about restoring balance and giving the body the conditions it needs to heal.

This case serves as further evidence that **when the Ten Natural Secrets in this book are applied consistently and comprehensively, meaningful improvements in blood sugar control are possible**, even in individuals with long-standing and medication-dependent diabetes.

A Biopsychosocial Approach to Reversing Diabetes

Diabetes is not a single-cause disease. It is a complex, progressive metabolic condition shaped by biological dysfunction, psychological stress, and lifestyle behaviors over time. For decades, diabetes management has focused primarily on blood sugar control through medications, while largely overlooking the interconnected systems that drive insulin resistance and metabolic breakdown. The result has been symptom management rather than true disease reversal. The ten natural secrets presented in this book are grounded in a biopsychosocial model of health. This model recognizes that chronic disease develops through the interaction of physiological processes, emotional and neurological regulation, and daily behaviors shaped by environment and culture. A growing body of scientific research supports this integrative framework, demonstrating that addressing diabetes at all three levels is essential for long-term metabolic recovery.

The Biopsychosocial Model Explained

The biopsychosocial model was first introduced by George Engel as a response to the limitations of the traditional biomedical model. Rather than viewing disease as a purely biological malfunction, this model recognizes that health and illness arise from the interaction of:

1. **Biological factors** such as insulin signaling, inflammation, hormonal balance, gut health, and nutrient status
2. **Psychological factors** including stress, trauma, anxiety, depression, and nervous system regulation
3. **Social and behavioral factors** such as diet, sleep, movement, medication use, environmental exposure, and daily habits

Diabetes exemplifies the need for this model. Insulin resistance is influenced not only by glucose intake, but also by cortisol, sleep deprivation, chronic inflammation, emotional stress, sedentary behavior, medication effects, and toxic exposure. Treating only blood sugar ignores the upstream drivers of disease progression.

1. Biological Evidence Supporting the 10 Secrets

Nutrition and Insulin Resistance

Dietary patterns are among the strongest predictors of insulin sensitivity. Diets high in refined carbohydrates, added sugars, and ultra-processed foods increase postprandial glucose spikes, promote chronic hyperinsulinemia, and accelerate beta-cell dysfunction. Large cohort studies have consistently shown that high glycemic load diets are associated with increased risk of type 2 diabetes (Hu et al., 2001). Conversely, whole-food, anti-inflammatory dietary patterns improve insulin sensitivity, reduce hepatic glucose production, and lower inflammatory markers. A systematic review published in *Diabetes Care* found that dietary interventions emphasizing whole foods significantly improved glycemic control independent of weight loss (Esposito et al., 2014).

Micronutrients and Metabolic Function

Multiple studies confirm that deficiencies in magnesium, vitamin D, zinc, chromium, and B vitamins impair insulin signaling and glucose metabolism. Magnesium deficiency, in particular, is strongly associated with insulin resistance and type 2 diabetes risk (Barbagallo & Dominguez, 2015). Vitamin D deficiency has been linked to impaired beta-cell function and increased inflammation (Pittas et al., 2010). Correcting these deficiencies through targeted, lab-guided intervention improves insulin sensitivity and metabolic outcomes, reinforcing the biological foundation of this approach.

Medications and Metabolic Dysfunction

Numerous medications including corticosteroids, antidepressants, statins, beta blockers, and certain antihypertensives have been shown to worsen insulin resistance and elevate fasting glucose levels. A large population-based study demonstrated that long-term corticosteroid use significantly increases diabetes incidence (Clore & Thurby-Hay, 2009). Deprescribing or appropriately modifying medication regimens under professional supervision has been shown to improve metabolic markers, underscoring the importance of addressing drug-induced contributors rather than layering additional medications.

2. Psychological Evidence: Stress, Trauma, and Blood Sugar

Stress and the HPA Axis

Chronic psychological stress activates the hypothalamic-pituitary-adrenal axis, increasing cortisol levels. Elevated cortisol promotes gluconeogenesis, inhibits insulin action, and increases visceral fat accumulation. Multiple studies have shown that individuals with chronic stress exhibit higher fasting glucose and insulin resistance independent of diet (Joseph & Golden, 2017). A longitudinal study published in *Psychosomatic Medicine* demonstrated that perceived stress significantly predicted the development of type 2 diabetes over time (Heraclides et al., 2009).

Anxiety, Depression, and Diabetes Risk

Depression and anxiety are independently associated with increased diabetes risk and poorer glycemic control. A meta-analysis involving over 300,000 participants found that depression increased the risk of developing type 2 diabetes by 60 percent (Mezuk et al., 2008). Neuroinflammation, disrupted sleep, altered appetite regulation, and reduced motivation for self-care all contribute to this relationship. Addressing mental health is therefore not optional, but foundational for metabolic recovery.

3. Behavioral and Social Evidence

Sleep Deprivation and Insulin Resistance

Sleep restriction impairs glucose tolerance and insulin sensitivity within days. Experimental studies have shown that even partial sleep deprivation reduces insulin sensitivity by up to 30 percent (Spiegel et al., 1999). Chronic sleep disruption alters leptin and ghrelin levels, increasing hunger and cravings for refined carbohydrates. Improving sleep duration and consistency has been shown to improve fasting glucose and insulin sensitivity (Tasali et al., 2014).

Physical Activity and Glucose Regulation

Regular physical activity enhances glucose uptake through insulin-independent pathways and improves mitochondrial efficiency. Meta-analyses confirm that moderate daily exercise significantly reduces HbA1c and improves insulin sensitivity even without weight loss (Umpierre et al., 2011). Importantly, consistency matters more than intensity, reinforcing the behavioral emphasis of this program.

Environmental Toxins and Endocrine Disruption

Exposure to endocrine-disrupting chemicals such as bisphenols, phthalates, and persistent organic pollutants has been linked to insulin resistance and diabetes. A review in *The Lancet Diabetes & Endocrinology* confirmed strong associations between toxin exposure and metabolic disease (Heindel et al., 2017). Reducing toxic load through behavioral and environmental changes improves metabolic resilience.

Why the 10 Secrets Must Be Addressed Together

Each of the ten natural secrets targets a distinct yet interconnected contributor to diabetes. Research consistently shows that single-intervention strategies produce limited results, while multi-component lifestyle interventions achieve superior and more durable outcomes. The Diabetes Prevention Program demonstrated that comprehensive lifestyle modification reduced diabetes incidence by 58 percent, outperforming medication alone (Knowler et al., 2002). This landmark trial underscores the necessity of addressing biology, psychology, and behavior simultaneously.

Conclusion: A Model Built on Science, Not Opinion

The approach outlined in this book is not experimental. It is aligned with decades of research across endocrinology, neuroscience, nutrition, psychology, and public health. The biopsychosocial model provides the missing framework needed to understand why diabetes persists despite medication escalation. Reversing diabetes requires correcting insulin resistance, calming the nervous system, restoring metabolic balance, and reshaping daily behaviors. Each of the ten natural secrets contributes to this process. Ignoring any one of them limits progress. This chapter establishes the scientific foundation for everything that follows. The chapters ahead translate this evidence into practical, step-by-step strategies that empower you to move from understanding to healing.

The Roadmap to Healing

If you are holding this book, it is likely because you are ready for something more than temporary solutions. You may be tired of managing blood sugar numbers without understanding why diabetes developed in the first place. You may feel frustrated by approaches that rely heavily on medication while leaving the root causes unaddressed. This book was written for you. It is designed to help you understand diabetes at its core and to guide you toward real, lasting metabolic healing.

Diabetes is not a random condition. In most cases, it develops slowly over time as a result of multiple overlapping factors, including diet, medications, chronic stress, nutrient deficiencies, hormonal imbalance, sleep disruption, environmental toxin exposure, and lifestyle habits. Conventional care often focuses on lowering blood glucose alone, but blood sugar is only one marker of a much deeper problem. To reverse diabetes safely and sustainably, the underlying dysfunction driving insulin resistance must be addressed.

Diabetes is a **complex, multifactorial condition**, which means there is no single cause and no single solution. This is why quick fixes and isolated interventions so often fail. True healing requires a comprehensive approach that restores balance across the entire metabolic system. That is the purpose of this book. This book presents **10 natural secrets**, each addressing a different contributor to diabetes. These secrets are not optional, interchangeable, or standalone strategies. They work together as an integrated system. Ignoring even one can limit progress and keep you trapped in cycles of blood sugar instability rather than achieving true reversal. When all ten are implemented together, they create the conditions the body needs to heal.

Each of these elements is explored in its own dedicated chapter. Every chapter explains **why that element matters**, **how it contributes to diabetes**, and **how to apply it step by step**. You will find clear guidance, practical strategies, and detailed plans designed to help you confidently execute each section in daily life. This structure ensures that you are not left guessing what to do next. Instead, you are given a clear, actionable roadmap to follow. Below is an overview of the 10 natural secrets that form the foundation of this healing process.

The 10 Natural Secrets to Reversing Diabetes

1. Food-Induced Diabetes

Food is one of the most powerful drivers of insulin resistance and blood sugar dysregulation. Diets high in refined carbohydrates, added sugars, processed foods, and inflammatory oils overload the pancreas and worsen metabolic dysfunction. Many individuals also unknowingly consume foods they are sensitive to, triggering immune responses that further impair insulin signaling. By removing inflammatory foods and adopting a nutrient-dense, anti-inflammatory eating pattern such as the ASTR Diet detailed in *Eat to Heal*, the body can begin restoring insulin sensitivity and metabolic balance.

2. Drug-Induced Diabetes

Many prescription and over-the-counter medications contribute to elevated blood sugar and insulin resistance. Steroids, statins, certain blood pressure medications, antidepressants, hormonal therapies, and other commonly used drugs can interfere with glucose metabolism. Identifying and addressing drug-induced contributors, in collaboration with a qualified healthcare provider, removes a major barrier to healing and allows the body to respond more effectively to lifestyle interventions.

3. Medicinal Teas

Medicinal teas provide gentle yet meaningful metabolic support. Teas such as green tea, oolong, rooibos, cinnamon, ginger, chamomile, and hibiscus contain compounds that improve insulin sensitivity, reduce oxidative stress, and support pancreatic function. While teas alone do not reverse diabetes, they serve as valuable daily allies when integrated into a comprehensive healing plan.

4. Vitamin, Mineral, and Hormonal Imbalances

Micronutrient deficiencies play a central role in diabetes and are frequently overlooked. Magnesium, chromium, zinc, vitamin D, and B-complex vitamins are essential for proper insulin signaling and glucose metabolism. Hormonal imbalances, including elevated cortisol and thyroid dysfunction, further impair blood sugar control. Identifying and correcting these imbalances is foundational to long-term metabolic healing.

5. Stress Management

Chronic stress keeps the body in a constant fight-or-flight state, driving cortisol elevations that raise blood sugar and worsen insulin resistance. Over time, stress contributes to inflammation, poor sleep, emotional eating, and metabolic exhaustion. Managing stress through nervous system regulation, mindfulness, prayer, breathing exercises, and emotional healing is a critical pillar of diabetes reversal.

6. Environmental Toxins

Environmental toxins interfere with hormonal signaling, mitochondrial function, and insulin sensitivity. Pesticides, plastics, heavy metals, and endocrine-

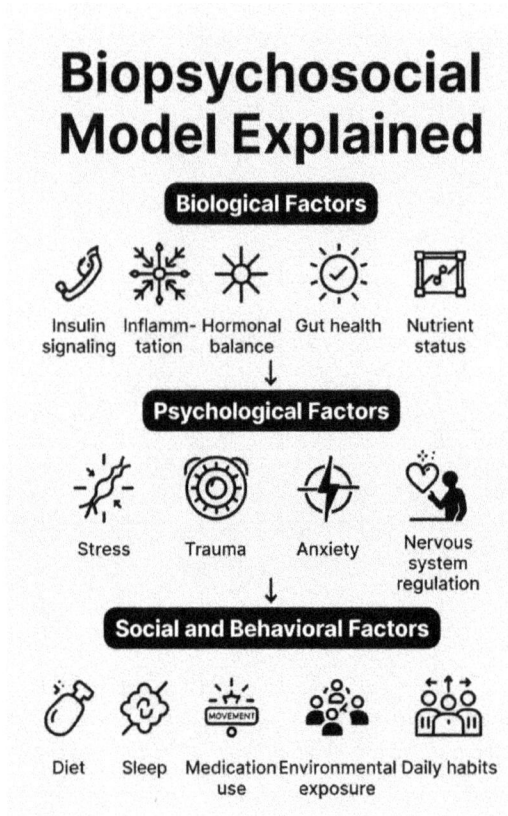

Biopsychosocial Model Explained

Biological Factors

Insulin signaling · Inflammation · Hormonal balance · Gut health · Nutrient status

Psychological Factors

Stress · Trauma · Anxiety · Nervous system regulation

Social and Behavioral Factors

Diet · Sleep · Medication use · Environmental exposure · Daily habits disrupting chemicals contribute silently to metabolic disease. Reducing toxic exposure through cleaner food, water, household products, and lifestyle choices removes an often-hidden obstacle to recovery.

7. Sleep

Sleep is one of the most underestimated factors in blood sugar regulation. Even short-term sleep deprivation significantly worsens insulin resistance. Restoring healthy sleep patterns improves hormone balance, appetite regulation, energy levels, and metabolic flexibility, making every other aspect of healing more effective.

8. Fasting

When applied correctly, fasting allows insulin levels to fall and gives the pancreas a break from constant stimulation. Strategic, individualized fasting supports metabolic flexibility and insulin sensitivity. This book presents fasting as a therapeutic tool, emphasizing safety, personalization, and sustainability rather than extremes.

9. Exercise

Movement increases glucose uptake and improves insulin sensitivity. Exercise does not need to be intense to be effective. Walking, resistance training, and consistent daily movement can significantly improve blood sugar control when performed regularly and appropriately.

10. Behavioral Modification

Lasting diabetes reversal requires lasting behavior change. Addressing habits such as emotional eating, sedentary routines, inconsistent sleep, and stress-driven coping patterns is essential. Small, consistent changes compound over time, creating a lifestyle that supports long-term metabolic health.

Why All 10 Secrets Matter

Diabetes does not develop from a single cause, and it cannot be reversed with a single solution. Each of these ten elements addresses a different contributor to the disease. Focusing on only one or two may produce short-term improvements, but true and lasting reversal requires addressing **all ten together**. This process is not about perfection. It is about progress. When these elements are implemented consistently and as a unified system, the body is given the opportunity to heal at the root.

Conclusion: Commit to the Full Path

Reversing diabetes is not about shortcuts. It is about addressing the real underlying causes with intention, consistency, and a comprehensive approach. These 10 natural secrets work together as an integrated system. Each one matters. Each one contributes. By committing to the full path, you are not simply managing a diagnosis. You are reclaiming your health at its foundation. As you move through the chapters that follow, you will gain the knowledge, tools, and confidence needed to take meaningful steps toward a healthier, more vibrant life.

Healing is possible. The roadmap is here. The next step is yours.

1. Food-Induced Diabetes

Diabetes does not begin with a diagnosis. It develops gradually, often over many years, as the body is repeatedly exposed to foods that disrupt blood sugar regulation, overwhelm insulin signaling, and promote chronic inflammation. While genetics may influence susceptibility, food remains one of the most powerful and modifiable contributors to insulin resistance and type 2 diabetes (Hu et al., 2001; Esposito et al., 2014). This chapter is not about fear or restriction. It is about understanding how specific foods affect your body and learning how to remove the obstacles that prevent healing. When the right foods are chosen and harmful triggers are identified, the body has a remarkable ability to restore metabolic balance.

How Food Drives Insulin Resistance

Every time you eat, your body must manage the rise in blood glucose that follows. In a healthy metabolic system, insulin efficiently moves glucose into cells for energy. When repeated blood sugar surges occur from highly processed or inflammatory foods, insulin is released in excessive amounts. Over time, cells become less responsive, leading to insulin resistance (DeFronzo & Tripathy, 2009). Insulin resistance is the core driver of type 2 diabetes. Long before blood glucose rises into the diabetic range, insulin levels are often chronically elevated. This state places continuous stress on the pancreas, promotes fat storage, worsens inflammation, and disrupts hormonal balance (Kahn et al., 2014). Food choices either accelerate this process or help reverse it.

Processed and Ultra-Processed Foods

Processed and ultra-processed foods are among the strongest contributors to insulin resistance. These foods are typically high in refined carbohydrates, added sugars, industrial seed oils, sodium, and chemical additives, while being low in fiber and essential nutrients. Ultra-processed foods rapidly elevate blood glucose and insulin, creating repeated metabolic stress. Large population studies have shown that higher consumption of ultra-processed foods is associated with a significantly increased risk of developing type 2 diabetes (Srour et al., 2020; Monteiro et al., 2019). These foods also displace nutrient-dense options, increasing the likelihood of deficiencies in magnesium, chromium, and potassium, which are essential for insulin signaling (Barbagallo &

Dominguez, 2015). Replacing processed foods with whole, minimally processed foods is one of the most effective ways to improve insulin sensitivity.

Refined Carbohydrates and Added Sugars

Refined carbohydrates and added sugars place a heavy burden on the pancreas. Foods such as white bread, pastries, cereals, desserts, and sugar-sweetened beverages are rapidly absorbed, leading to sharp spikes in blood glucose followed by large insulin surges. Over time, this pattern drives insulin resistance and beta cell fatigue (Ludwig, 2002). High-glycemic diets have been consistently linked to increased risk of type 2 diabetes, even in individuals who are not overweight (Salmerón et al., 1997). Excess fructose intake, particularly from high-fructose corn syrup, further worsens insulin resistance by promoting fatty liver, increasing uric acid levels, and impairing glucose metabolism (Johnson et al., 2007). Reducing refined carbohydrates and added sugars while prioritizing fiber-rich whole foods allows insulin levels to fall and metabolic flexibility to improve.

Industrial Seed Oils and Inflammatory Fats

Industrial seed oils such as soybean, corn, canola, sunflower, and safflower oils are widely used in processed foods and restaurant meals. These oils are high in omega-6 fatty acids, which promote inflammation when consumed in excess. Chronic inflammation interferes with insulin signaling and worsens metabolic health (Hotamisligil, 2006). Diets high in omega-6 fats relative to omega-3 fats have been associated with increased insulin resistance and oxidative stress (Simopoulos, 2016). Replacing inflammatory oils with more stable fats such as olive oil supports improved insulin sensitivity and metabolic health.

Alcohol

Alcohol significantly disrupts glucose metabolism. The liver must prioritize detoxifying alcohol over regulating blood sugar, which interferes with glucose control and promotes fat accumulation in the liver. Regular alcohol consumption has been associated with increased insulin resistance and higher risk of type 2 diabetes (Knott et al., 2015). Large global analyses have concluded that **no level of alcohol consumption is truly safe** for long-term health (GBD 2018 Alcohol

Collaborators, 2018). Eliminating alcohol reduces metabolic strain and supports liver and pancreatic recovery.

Artificial Sweeteners

Artificial sweeteners are often marketed as diabetes-friendly alternatives to sugar, yet research suggests they may worsen glucose tolerance in some individuals. Studies show that artificial sweeteners can alter gut microbiota and disrupt metabolic signaling, contributing to insulin resistance (Suez et al., 2014). Despite containing no calories, these compounds may confuse the body's glucose regulation systems and promote blood sugar instability. Limiting artificial sweeteners supports more stable glycemic control.

Additives and Preservatives

Food additives such as emulsifiers, preservatives, and flavor enhancers are increasingly recognized as contributors to metabolic dysfunction. These compounds can disrupt gut barrier integrity, increase inflammation, and impair insulin signaling (Chassaing et al., 2015). Processed and preserved foods often contain combinations of additives that create cumulative metabolic stress. Choosing foods with simple, recognizable ingredients reduces exposure to these hidden contributors.

Dairy and Casein Sensitivity

Some individuals experience inflammatory responses to pasteurized dairy products, particularly casein proteins. Heat processing alters protein structure, increasing immune reactivity in susceptible individuals (Jianqin et al., 2016). Chronic low-grade inflammation driven by food sensitivities can worsen insulin resistance. Some individuals tolerate fermented, raw, goat, or sheep dairy better than conventional pasteurized cow dairy, while others benefit from eliminating dairy entirely.

Dehydration and Electrolyte Imbalance

Hydration plays a critical role in glucose regulation. Dehydration increases stress hormone release and worsens insulin resistance (Kenney & Chiu, 2001).

Electrolytes such as magnesium and potassium are essential for insulin signaling and glucose transport. Magnesium deficiency is common in people with diabetes and is associated with impaired insulin sensitivity (Barbagallo & Dominguez, 2015). Adequate hydration and mineral intake through whole foods support metabolic stability.

Excessive Protein From Processed Sources

Protein is essential for metabolic health, but excessive intake from processed sources such as protein bars, powders, and processed meats can undermine blood sugar control. Many of these products contain hidden sugars, artificial sweeteners, and additives that worsen insulin resistance. Whole-food protein sources support stable glucose regulation without unnecessary metabolic stress.

Food Sensitivities and Immune Activation

Food sensitivities can quietly drive inflammation, stress hormone release, and insulin resistance. Unlike immediate allergic reactions, sensitivities may present as fatigue, cravings, digestive discomfort, brain fog, or unstable blood sugar (Jackson et al., 2018). Identifying and eliminating personal food triggers can significantly improve insulin sensitivity and metabolic outcomes.

How to Identify Your Personal Food Triggers for Diabetes

Because diabetes is influenced by individualized factors, it is essential to systematically identify which foods contribute to blood sugar instability and insulin resistance. Most people have more than three dietary triggers. The goal is clarity, not perfection.

Keep a Detailed Food, Glucose, and Symptom Journal

Tracking food intake, timing, blood glucose before and after meals, and symptoms such as fatigue, cravings, shakiness, headaches, or brain fog helps reveal patterns. Sleep, stress, hydration, and physical activity should also be recorded.

Use an ASTR Diet Elimination Strategy

1. Food-Induced Diabetes

The ASTR Diet helps identify and remove food-induced diabetes triggers through an anti-inflammatory, toxin-free, and restorative approach. Common triggers are removed temporarily, then reintroduced systematically while monitoring blood glucose and symptoms. Detailed guidance is provided in *Eat to Heal* Book.

Test Foods Individually

Some individuals prefer to test foods one at a time. Blood glucose should be measured before and one to two hours after eating. Foods that consistently cause glucose spikes or symptoms should be avoided.

Be Cautious When Testing Dairy

Dairy reactions vary widely. Small amounts should be tested, with attention to differences between milk, cheese, and yogurt. Some individuals tolerate goat or sheep dairy better than cow dairy, while others benefit from a longer dairy-free trial.

Conclusion: How Food-Induced Diabetes Fits Into the 10 Natural Secrets

Food is often the first place diabetes begins and the first place meaningful healing can occur. The dietary patterns discussed in this chapter directly influence insulin resistance, inflammation, and metabolic stress, which are central drivers of diabetes. Addressing food-induced contributors lays the groundwork for every other natural secret in this book to work more effectively.

When inflammatory foods, refined carbohydrates, added sugars, and individual food sensitivities are removed, insulin demand decreases and metabolic flexibility improves. This creates a more responsive internal environment for the strategies covered in the surrounding chapters, including medication review, nutrient repletion, fasting, movement, stress regulation, sleep restoration, toxin reduction, and behavioral change.Food alone, however, is rarely the entire story. Diabetes is complex, and dietary change must be paired with the other natural secrets to achieve lasting results. When food is addressed as part of a comprehensive, integrated approach, it becomes a powerful tool not only for stabilizing blood sugar, but for restoring the body's natural ability to heal.

1. Food-Induced Diabetes

Because diet is the foundation of blood sugar control, proper food choices and meal timing are essential for reversing diabetes. However, it is not possible to fully cover the depth and structure of a therapeutic diet within the scope of this book without oversimplifying a process that requires precision and consistency. For this reason, the nutritional strategy used alongside the principles in this book is explained in detail in *Eat to Heal*, which outlines how to choose anti-inflammatory, nutrient-dense foods, structure meals to stabilize blood sugar, and implement sustainable eating rhythms that support metabolic healing. Most importantly, *Eat to Heal* breaks down this approach into clear, practical steps, making it easy to integrate into daily life without extreme restriction, confusion, or short-term dieting, allowing readers to apply these principles consistently for long-term blood sugar stability and true metabolic restoration.

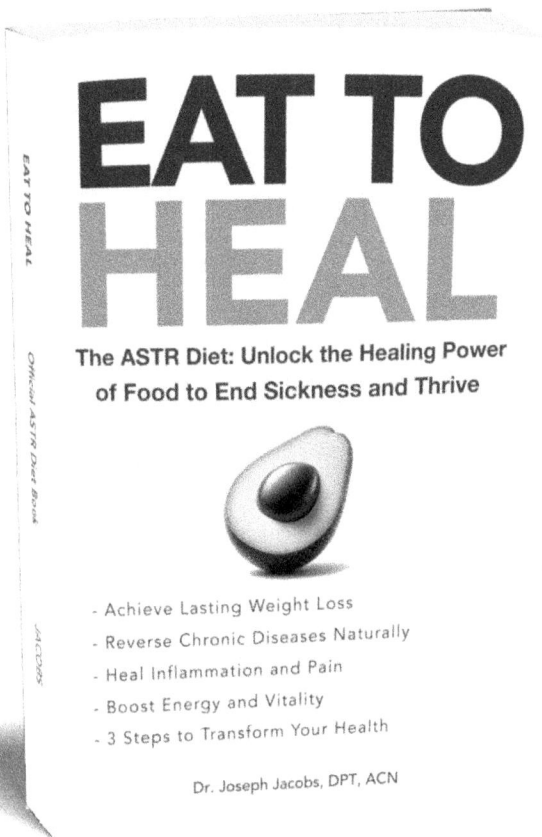

EAT TO HEAL

EAT TO HEAL

Official ASTR Diet Book

JACOBS

The ASTR Diet: Unlock the Healing Power of Food to End Sickness and Thrive

- Achieve Lasting Weight Loss
- Reverse Chronic Diseases Naturally
- Heal Inflammation and Pain
- Boost Energy and Vitality
- 3 Steps to Transform Your Health

Dr. Joseph Jacobs, DPT, ACN

2. Drug-Induced Diabetes

Diabetes is often viewed as a condition driven primarily by diet and lifestyle, yet medications are an overlooked and significant contributor to insulin resistance and blood sugar dysregulation. Many commonly prescribed and over-the-counter drugs can impair glucose metabolism, elevate insulin levels, and accelerate the progression toward type 2 diabetes. In some cases, medication use may be the primary factor preventing blood sugar from improving despite diligent dietary and lifestyle changes.

Understanding how medications influence metabolic health is essential, particularly for individuals seeking to reverse diabetes rather than simply manage it. This chapter reviews classes of medications commonly associated with drug-induced diabetes, the mechanisms through which they disrupt glucose regulation, and the importance of addressing these contributors as part of a comprehensive healing plan.

1. Corticosteroids

Corticosteroids are among the most well-documented medications associated with drug-induced diabetes. These medications are commonly prescribed for asthma, autoimmune disorders, allergic reactions, inflammatory conditions, joint pain, and skin disorders. While they can provide rapid symptom relief, corticosteroids significantly impair glucose metabolism.

Corticosteroids raise blood sugar by increasing hepatic glucose production and reducing insulin sensitivity in peripheral tissues. They also promote fat redistribution, muscle breakdown, and appetite stimulation, all of which contribute to worsening insulin resistance. Even short-term use can cause significant hyperglycemia, particularly in individuals with underlying metabolic vulnerability. A large cohort study found that chronic corticosteroid use was associated with a markedly increased risk of developing type 2 diabetes, with risk rising as dose and duration increased (Clore & Thurby-Hay, 2009). Long-term exposure places continuous stress on pancreatic beta cells and may hasten the need for glucose-lowering medications. For individuals requiring corticosteroids, using the lowest effective dose for the shortest duration possible is critical. Close monitoring of blood glucose and insulin levels is essential during therapy.

2. Statins

Statins are widely prescribed to lower cholesterol. Multiple large studies have demonstrated an association between statin use and increased risk of developing diabetes. Statins may impair insulin sensitivity by interfering with glucose transport into muscle cells and altering pancreatic beta cell function. They may also promote mild weight gain and increase insulin resistance over time. A meta-analysis of randomized controlled trials found that statin therapy was associated with a significant increase in new-onset diabetes, particularly in individuals with preexisting metabolic risk factors (Sattar et al., 2010). For patients experiencing rising blood sugar or worsening insulin resistance while on statins, alternative strategies should be explored.

3. Antidepressants

Antidepressants are commonly prescribed for depression, anxiety, chronic pain, and sleep disorders. Certain classes are associated with impaired glucose regulation and increased diabetes risk. Tricyclic antidepressants and some serotonin norepinephrine reuptake inhibitors can worsen insulin resistance by increasing sympathetic nervous system activity and altering cortisol regulation. Weight gain and appetite changes associated with antidepressant use further compound metabolic risk. A population-based study found that long-term antidepressant use was associated with an increased incidence of type 2 diabetes (Pan et al., 2012). Selective serotonin reuptake inhibitors may have a more neutral metabolic profile for some individuals, but blood glucose monitoring is still recommended, particularly with long-term use or combination therapy.

4. Antipsychotic Medications

Second-generation antipsychotics are strongly associated with metabolic dysfunction. Medications such as olanzapine, clozapine, quetiapine, and risperidone significantly increase the risk of insulin resistance, weight gain, and type 2 diabetes. These drugs impair insulin signaling, increase appetite, and alter lipid metabolism. In some cases, profound hyperglycemia can develop within weeks of initiation. A large observational study demonstrated a significantly higher incidence of diabetes among individuals taking atypical antipsychotics compared with the general population (Newcomer, 2005).

5. Oral Contraceptives and Hormonal Therapies

Hormonal medications, including oral contraceptives and hormone replacement therapy, can influence insulin sensitivity and glucose regulation. Estrogen and progestins affect hepatic glucose production and may promote insulin resistance in susceptible individuals. Long-term use has been associated with changes in glucose tolerance, particularly in women with underlying metabolic risk factors such as polycystic ovary syndrome, obesity, or family history of diabetes. Monitoring blood glucose and insulin markers is important for women using hormonal therapies (Godsland, 2005).

6. Stimulant Medications

Stimulants prescribed for attention deficit hyperactivity disorder, narcolepsy, and fatigue increase sympathetic nervous system activity. These medications raise cortisol and adrenaline levels, which promote insulin resistance and blood sugar elevation. Amphetamines and methylphenidate may cause appetite suppression initially, but chronic use can disrupt glucose regulation and stress hormonal balance. Over-the-counter stimulants, including caffeine-heavy energy drinks and weight loss supplements, may further amplify metabolic strain. Addressing underlying contributors to fatigue, such as nutrient deficiencies, sleep disruption, and blood sugar instability, may reduce reliance on stimulant medications.

7. Immunosuppressive Medications

Immunosuppressive drugs used for autoimmune diseases and organ transplantation can significantly impair glucose metabolism. Calcineurin inhibitors such as tacrolimus and cyclosporine interfere with insulin secretion and increase insulin resistance. Studies show a high incidence of post-transplant diabetes among patients receiving these medications (Vincenti et al., 2007). Corticosteroids used alongside immunosuppressants further compound metabolic dysfunction. Careful monitoring and supportive metabolic strategies are essential for individuals requiring immunosuppressive therapy.

8. Chemotherapy and Targeted Cancer Therapies

Certain chemotherapy agents and targeted cancer therapies increase the risk of insulin resistance and diabetes. These drugs may damage pancreatic beta cells, increase oxidative stress, and disrupt hormonal regulation. Targeted therapies that interfere with growth signaling pathways can impair glucose metabolism and contribute to persistent hyperglycemia. Survivors of cancer treatment may experience long-term metabolic consequences, making post-treatment monitoring critical (Choueiri et al., 2010).

Why Addressing Drug-Induced Diabetes Matters

When medications contribute to insulin resistance, dietary changes alone may not be enough to restore metabolic health. Many individuals become discouraged when blood sugar fails to improve despite significant lifestyle effort. In these cases, medication review is a crucial and often missing step. This does not mean medications should be stopped abruptly or without medical supervision. Rather, it highlights the importance of working with knowledgeable professionals who understand both metabolic health and medication physiology.

Conclusion: How Drug-Induced Diabetes Fits Into the 10 Natural Secrets

Medication-induced insulin resistance is one of the most overlooked barriers to reversing diabetes. As explored in this chapter, many commonly prescribed and over-the-counter medications can impair glucose metabolism, elevate insulin levels, and counteract even the most consistent dietary and lifestyle efforts. When progress stalls despite genuine commitment to change, medications are often a hidden but significant contributor.

Addressing drug-induced diabetes strengthens the effectiveness of every other natural secret in this book. When medications that worsen insulin resistance are identified and appropriately managed, the body becomes more responsive to nutritional therapy, fasting strategies, nutrient repletion, exercise, stress regulation, sleep restoration, toxin reduction, and behavioral change.

For this reason, it is essential to work with an **advanced clinical nutritionist and a healthcare provider who is educated in metabolic health, medication effects, and safe deprescribing strategies**. With proper guidance, it is often possible to reduce, replace, or eliminate medications that worsen insulin resistance and transition to safer alternatives while supporting the body's natural ability to heal. This chapter reinforces a central principle of diabetes reversal. Healing is not about adding more interventions, but about removing the obstacles that prevent recovery. When medication burden is addressed as part of a comprehensive, integrated approach, the full roadmap of the 10 Natural Secrets can work together to restore balance and promote lasting metabolic health.

3. Medicinal Teas

Medicinal teas have been used for centuries across cultures to support metabolic health, reduce inflammation, and restore balance within the body. While often viewed as gentle or supportive remedies, growing research shows that certain teas can meaningfully improve insulin sensitivity, stabilize blood sugar, and reduce oxidative stress. When used consistently and intentionally, medicinal teas can serve as a valuable component of a comprehensive diabetes reversal strategy.

Medicinal teas are not intended to replace foundational interventions such as nutrition, movement, medication review, or stress management. Instead, they function as supportive tools that enhance the body's healing environment and reinforce metabolic regulation. This chapter explores specific teas that have demonstrated benefits for glucose control and insulin resistance, supported by scientific evidence and clinical observation.

How Medicinal Teas Support Blood Sugar Regulation

Medicinal teas influence metabolic health through multiple pathways. Many contain polyphenols and flavonoids that improve insulin sensitivity, protect pancreatic beta cells from oxidative damage, and reduce systemic inflammation. Others support liver detoxification, slow carbohydrate absorption, and positively influence gut microbiota, all of which play critical roles in glucose regulation. When consumed regularly, certain teas have been associated with improvements in fasting glucose, reductions in postprandial glucose spikes, and lower markers of insulin resistance. Their effectiveness depends on consistency, appropriate selection, and integration into a broader healing plan.

Green Tea

Green tea is one of the most extensively studied medicinal teas for metabolic health. It contains catechins, particularly epigallocatechin gallate, which improve insulin sensitivity and reduce inflammation. These compounds enhance glucose uptake in skeletal muscle and reduce hepatic glucose production. Population studies have shown that regular green tea consumption is associated with lower fasting glucose levels and a reduced risk of developing type 2 diabetes (Huxley et al., 2009). Green tea also supports weight regulation and cardiovascular health, making it particularly beneficial for individuals with insulin resistance. For those sensitive to caffeine, lower caffeine varieties or earlier daytime consumption may be better tolerated.

Oolong Tea

Oolong tea, which is partially oxidized, offers unique metabolic benefits. Research suggests that oolong tea improves glucose metabolism by enhancing insulin sensitivity and reducing post meal glucose excursions. A clinical study demonstrated that daily consumption of oolong tea significantly reduced fasting blood glucose levels in individuals with type 2 diabetes (Hosoda et al., 2003). Oolong tea may be especially helpful for individuals who experience elevated blood sugar after meals.

Black Tea

Black tea contains theaflavins and thearubigins, antioxidant compounds that reduce oxidative stress and inflammation. These compounds have been shown to support insulin sensitivity and glucose metabolism. Epidemiological studies indicate that black tea consumption is associated with improved metabolic health and lower diabetes risk (InterAct Consortium, 2012). Black tea may also support vascular health, which is particularly important given the increased cardiovascular risk associated with diabetes.

Hibiscus Tea

Hibiscus tea is rich in anthocyanins and polyphenols that support metabolic and vascular function. While commonly studied for blood pressure regulation, hibiscus also demonstrates benefits for insulin sensitivity and oxidative stress reduction. Clinical studies suggest that hibiscus tea may lower fasting glucose levels and improve lipid profiles, both of which are important in diabetes management (Mozaffari-Khosravi et al., 2014). Its caffeine free nature makes it suitable for regular consumption throughout the day.

Rooibos Tea

Rooibos tea is a naturally caffeine free herbal tea rich in antioxidants, including aspalathin. Aspalathin has been shown to improve glucose uptake and reduce insulin resistance in experimental studies. Research suggests that rooibos supports pancreatic beta cell function and reduces oxidative stress associated with diabetes (Kawano et al., 2009). Rooibos is well tolerated and can be consumed in the evening without affecting sleep.

Cinnamon Tea

Cinnamon has long been recognized for its role in blood sugar regulation. Cinnamon tea provides a gentle method of delivering bioactive compounds that improve insulin sensitivity and slow gastric emptying. Clinical studies demonstrate that cinnamon supplementation can lower fasting glucose and improve insulin sensitivity in individuals with type 2 diabetes (Khan et al., 2003). Cinnamon tea may be particularly useful for managing post meal glucose elevations.

Ginger Tea

Ginger tea supports glucose regulation by reducing inflammation and improving insulin sensitivity. Ginger also supports digestive function, which can influence glucose absorption and insulin response. A randomized controlled trial found that ginger supplementation significantly reduced fasting blood glucose and hemoglobin A1C levels in individuals with type 2 diabetes (Mahluji et al., 2013). Ginger tea provides a warming, caffeine free option that supports metabolic health.

Chamomile Tea

Chamomile tea supports glucose regulation indirectly by calming the nervous system and improving sleep quality. Chronic stress and poor sleep elevate cortisol levels, which worsen insulin resistance. Animal and early human studies suggest chamomile may reduce blood glucose and oxidative stress markers (Kato et al., 2008). Chamomile is particularly beneficial when consumed in the evening as part of a bedtime routine.

Peppermint and Lemon Balm Tea

Peppermint and lemon balm teas support digestive health and nervous system balance. Improved digestion and reduced stress can positively influence glucose regulation. Lemon balm has demonstrated antioxidant and glucose lowering effects in experimental studies (Weidner et al., 2015). These teas are gentle, widely tolerated, and useful as supportive daily options.

How to Use Medicinal Teas Effectively

Medicinal teas are most effective when consumed consistently rather than occasionally. One to three cups per day is generally sufficient, depending on the type of tea and individual tolerance. Teas should be consumed without added sugar or artificial sweeteners, as these undermine metabolic benefits. Rotating teas can provide a broader range of beneficial compounds while reducing reliance on any single herb. Individuals sensitive to caffeine should prioritize herbal teas or limit caffeinated varieties to earlier in the day. Medicinal teas should be viewed as supportive tools, not standalone treatments. Their benefits are maximized when combined with proper nutrition, movement, stress regulation, medication review, and adequate sleep.

Conclusion: How Medicinal Teas Fit Into the 10 Natural Secrets

Medicinal teas reinforce the work done in the earlier chapters by supporting insulin sensitivity, reducing inflammation, and calming the nervous system. They complement the foundational role of food by enhancing metabolic stability, support the medication review process by easing metabolic stress, and work synergistically with stress management and sleep optimization. Like every natural secret presented in this book, medicinal teas are not meant to function in isolation. Their greatest impact occurs when they are integrated with the other elements of the program, including nutrition, nutrient balance, fasting, movement, behavioral change, toxin reduction, and restorative sleep.

Diabetes is a complex condition that requires a comprehensive approach. Medicinal teas provide gentle but meaningful support that helps the body respond more effectively to the other interventions you are implementing. When used consistently alongside the full roadmap, they become an ally in restoring balance and moving the body toward lasting metabolic healing.

4. Vitamin, Mineral, and Hormonal Imbalances

Diabetes is not merely a disorder of elevated blood glucose. It is a complex metabolic condition driven by insulin resistance, chronic inflammation, oxidative stress, and impaired cellular signaling. While dietary patterns and lifestyle behaviors are foundational to diabetes reversal, vitamin, mineral, and hormonal imbalances often determine whether meaningful healing can occur. Without identifying and correcting these underlying deficiencies, many individuals struggle to improve insulin sensitivity or achieve stable blood sugar control.

Clinical and epidemiological research consistently demonstrates that individuals with diabetes exhibit multiple micronutrient and hormonal deficiencies that impair glucose metabolism (Pittas et al., 2010; Guerrero-Romero et al., 2011). From my clinical experience, most patients with diabetes present with **four to eight concurrent deficiencies**, each contributing to insulin resistance and metabolic dysfunction. Because biochemical needs vary widely, **laboratory-guided, individualized care is essential**. Supplementation without proper testing is not only ineffective but potentially harmful.

Vitamin D Deficiency

Vitamin D plays a critical role in insulin secretion, insulin sensitivity, and immune regulation. Vitamin D receptors are expressed in pancreatic beta cells, skeletal muscle, and adipose tissue, all of which are involved in glucose metabolism. Low serum vitamin D levels are strongly associated with insulin resistance and increased risk of type 2 diabetes (Pittas et al., 2010). A meta-analysis of randomized controlled trials found that vitamin D supplementation improved insulin sensitivity and fasting glucose in individuals with baseline deficiency (Seida et al., 2014). However, supplementation must be guided by laboratory testing. Excessive vitamin D intake may cause hypercalcemia, kidney stones, vascular calcification, nausea, and cardiac rhythm disturbances. Serum 25-hydroxyvitamin D levels should be monitored regularly to ensure safe and effective dosing.

Magnesium Deficiency

Magnesium is essential for insulin receptor signaling, glucose transport, and cellular energy production. Individuals with diabetes often experience increased urinary magnesium loss, making deficiency common (Guerrero-Romero &

Rodríguez-Morán, 2011). A meta-analysis of randomized trials demonstrated that magnesium supplementation significantly improved fasting glucose, insulin sensitivity, and HbA1c levels in individuals with type 2 diabetes (Simental-Mendía et al., 2016). Despite its benefits, unsupervised magnesium supplementation may cause diarrhea, hypotension, confusion, cardiac arrhythmias, and kidney dysfunction. Because serum magnesium may not reflect intracellular status, advanced testing is often required.

Vitamin B12 Deficiency

Vitamin B12 is essential for nerve integrity, methylation, and red blood cell formation. Deficiency is especially common in individuals taking metformin, a first-line diabetes medication known to impair B12 absorption (Reinstatler et al., 2012). Low B12 levels are associated with worsening insulin resistance and diabetic neuropathy. Long-term deficiency can cause irreversible nerve damage. Supplementation without proper assessment may mask other deficiencies or cause neurological symptoms such as numbness, itching, anxiety, or headaches. Personalized dosing based on laboratory evaluation is essential.

Vitamin B6 Deficiency

Vitamin B6 supports amino acid metabolism, neurotransmitter synthesis, and homocysteine regulation. Deficiency has been associated with increased oxidative stress and impaired glucose metabolism (Verhoef et al., 2002). While supplementation may support insulin sensitivity, excessive intake without guidance may cause sensory neuropathy, numbness, and tingling, which is particularly concerning in individuals already at risk for diabetic nerve damage. Personalized dosing based on laboratory evaluation is essential.

Folate (Vitamin B9) Deficiency

Folate plays a central role in methylation and DNA synthesis. Low folate status contributes to elevated homocysteine levels, endothelial dysfunction, and impaired insulin signaling (Forman et al., 2005). Folate supplementation may improve insulin sensitivity, particularly in individuals with MTHFR polymorphisms. However, excessive folate intake can mask vitamin B12 deficiency and worsen neurological outcomes. Genetic and biochemical testing should guide both form and dosage.

Iron Imbalance

Iron status significantly influences insulin sensitivity. Both iron deficiency and iron overload impair glucose metabolism. Elevated ferritin levels are strongly associated with insulin resistance and increased diabetes risk (Fernández-Real et al., 2002). Conversely, iron deficiency anemia impairs mitochondrial function and glucose utilization. Supplementation without laboratory confirmation may cause liver toxicity, oxidative stress, joint pain, gastrointestinal distress, and cardiovascular complications. Ferritin, transferrin saturation, and hemoglobin levels must be assessed before intervention.

Zinc Deficiency

Zinc is required for insulin synthesis, storage, and secretion. Deficiency impairs pancreatic beta-cell function and increases oxidative stress. A systematic review demonstrated that zinc supplementation significantly improved fasting glucose and HbA1c levels in individuals with diabetes (Jayawardena et al., 2012). Excess zinc intake without monitoring may cause copper deficiency, immune suppression, nausea, and hormonal imbalance. Supplementation must be individualized and carefully monitored.

Chromium Deficiency

Chromium enhances insulin receptor signaling and glucose uptake. Deficiency has been associated with impaired glucose tolerance and insulin resistance (Anderson et al., 1997). While chromium supplementation may benefit deficient individuals, inappropriate use has been linked to kidney and liver toxicity. Chromium should only be used after laboratory confirmation and under professional supervision.

Thyroid Hormone Imbalances

Thyroid hormones regulate basal metabolic rate, glucose utilization, and insulin sensitivity. Hypothyroidism, including subclinical forms, is associated with increased insulin resistance and poor glycemic control (Udovcic et al., 2017). Comprehensive thyroid testing, including TSH, free T3, free T4, and thyroid antibodies, is critical when diabetes is difficult to manage. Improper hormone supplementation may worsen blood sugar instability, cause arrhythmias, and disrupt adrenal function.

Cortisol Dysregulation

Cortisol directly raises blood glucose by stimulating gluconeogenesis and inhibiting insulin action. Chronic stress, sleep disruption, and adrenal dysfunction lead to persistently elevated cortisol levels, worsening insulin resistance (Whitworth et al., 2005). Addressing cortisol imbalance through testing, stress reduction, and targeted interventions is essential. Attempting adrenal support without evaluation may worsen anxiety, fatigue, sleep disturbances, and blood sugar volatility.

Conclusion: How Nutrient and Hormonal Balance Fits Into the 10 Natural Secrets

Vitamin, mineral, and hormonal imbalances are among the most powerful yet overlooked drivers of diabetes. Nutrition, fasting, exercise, and stress management cannot fully restore metabolic health if the biochemical foundations required for insulin signaling are compromised. For this reason, it is essential to work with a **clinical nutritionist trained in metabolic and functional medicine** who can identify deficiencies through comprehensive laboratory testing and determine the safest and most effective nutrient forms and dosages. **Supplementation without guidance is not safe** and may worsen insulin resistance or create new imbalances. When nutrient repletion and hormonal optimization are addressed alongside the other natural secrets in this book, including food, medication review, fasting, movement, sleep, stress regulation, toxin reduction, and behavioral change, the body becomes capable of true metabolic restoration. Diabetes reversal requires precision, integration, and professional guidance. When these elements work together, lasting healing becomes possible.

5. Exercise

Exercise for Lowering Blood Sugar

Regular physical activity is one of the most effective natural strategies for lowering blood sugar and improving insulin sensitivity. Consistent exercise helps muscles absorb glucose more efficiently, reduces insulin resistance, improves mitochondrial function, lowers systemic inflammation, and supports hormonal balance, all of which are critical for reversing diabetes. The American Heart Association recommends at least 150 minutes of moderate-intensity physical activity per week. This level of consistent movement has been shown to significantly improve blood sugar control, insulin sensitivity, and overall metabolic health (Pescatello et al., 2015).

Benefits of Exercise for Blood Sugar Control

- **Improved Insulin Sensitivity:** Exercise increases glucose uptake by skeletal muscle independent of insulin, allowing blood sugar levels to decrease more efficiently (Ross et al., 2000).
- **Improved Glucose Utilization:** Physical activity enhances the body's ability to use glucose for energy rather than storing it as fat, reducing post-meal blood sugar spikes.
- **Weight and Fat Mass Reduction:** Even modest reductions in visceral fat significantly improve insulin signaling and glycemic control (Stevens et al., 2001).
- **Stress Reduction:** Exercise lowers cortisol and improves nervous system regulation. Chronic stress and elevated cortisol are well-known contributors to blood sugar dysregulation (Paluska & Schwenk, 2000).
- **Improved Muscle Mass:** Increased lean muscle mass improves long-term glucose disposal and metabolic flexibility, a key factor in diabetes reversal.

Types of Exercises That Help Lower Blood Sugar

Several forms of exercise have been shown to significantly improve blood sugar control and insulin sensitivity, many of which can be done at home without special equipment.

1. Aerobic Exercise

Examples: Brisk walking, jogging in place, dancing, stair climbing, stationary cycling
Benefits: Improves insulin sensitivity and lowers fasting and post-meal blood sugar by increasing glucose uptake into muscle cells (Cornelissen & Fagard, 2005).
At-Home Tip: Aim for 30 minutes of brisk walking or dancing daily, especially after meals to blunt glucose spikes.

2. Resistance Training

Examples: Bodyweight exercises (squats, lunges, push-ups), resistance bands
Benefits: Builds muscle mass, which increases basal glucose utilization and improves insulin sensitivity (MacDonald et al., 2016).
At-Home Tip: Perform 2–3 sets of 10–15 repetitions of major muscle group exercises, 2–3 times per week.

3. Isometric Exercises

Examples: Wall sits, plank holds, handgrip exercises
Benefits: Improves metabolic efficiency and insulin response while placing minimal strain on joints, making it suitable for beginners or individuals with limited mobility (Inder et al., 2016).
At-Home Tip: Try 1–2 minute wall sits or plank holds several times per week.

4. Mind-Body Exercises

Examples: Yoga, tai chi, controlled breathing
Benefits: Reduce cortisol, improve autonomic balance, and support blood sugar regulation by calming stress-driven glucose release from the liver (Cui et al., 2016).
At-Home Tip: Incorporate 10–20 minutes of gentle yoga or guided breathing daily.

A Simple Way to Lower Blood Sugar While You Sit

Using an **under-desk bike** or seated **elliptical** is a simple and effective way to improve blood sugar control throughout the day. Light, continuous movement helps muscles pull glucose from the bloodstream, reducing post-meal spikes and improving insulin sensitivity, even at low intensity. These devices are especially useful for individuals who sit for long periods, work at a desk, or have limited mobility. Regular use can meaningfully improve blood sugar levels, circulation, and metabolic health without requiring structured workout sessions. I often recommend this type of movement for older adults, individuals with joint pain, or those who cannot tolerate prolonged walking. Start with 5–10 minutes per day and gradually increase to 30–45 minutes. This low-impact approach makes consistent movement achievable and sustainable, which is essential for reversing diabetes.

Exercise Timing and Blood Sugar Stability

The timing of exercise influences its impact on blood sugar. For many individuals with diabetes, **light to moderate exercise after meals** is particularly effective for lowering postprandial glucose. A study published in *Diabetes Care* found that walking after meals significantly reduced blood sugar compared to remaining sedentary (DiPietro et al., 2013). Fasted exercise may benefit some individuals, but in others it can raise stress hormones and worsen glucose variability. Timing should be individualized.

Safety Considerations for Diabetes Patients

Exercise directly affects blood glucose, insulin needs, hydration, and electrolyte balance. Individuals with diabetes should approach exercise with awareness and appropriate medical guidance. Important considerations include:

• Monitoring blood glucose before and after exercise
• Preventing hypoglycemia
• Adjusting medications when needed
• Supporting hydration and electrolytes
• Choosing joint-safe movements

Those with neuropathy, retinopathy, cardiovascular disease, or balance issues require individualized exercise plans.

Tips

- Start gradually and consult a healthcare provider if you have underlying medical conditions.
- Maintain hydration and proper form to avoid injury.
- Combine aerobic, resistance, and stress-reducing movement for optimal blood sugar control.

Conclusion: How Exercise Fits Into the 10 Natural Secrets

Exercise reinforces the work done in the earlier chapters by improving insulin sensitivity, increasing glucose uptake by muscle tissue, reducing inflammation, and regulating the nervous system. It strengthens the foundation established through proper nutrition and meal timing, supports medication review and deprescribing efforts by lowering metabolic demand, and works synergistically with stress reduction and sleep optimization to stabilize blood sugar levels. Like every natural secret presented in this book, exercise is not intended to function in isolation. Its greatest impact occurs when it is integrated with the full program, including nutrient balance, fasting strategies, behavioral change, toxin reduction, and restorative sleep.

Diabetes is a complex metabolic condition that requires a comprehensive, systems-based approach. Exercise provides a powerful and accessible stimulus that helps the body respond more effectively to all other interventions being implemented. When practiced consistently and appropriately alongside the complete roadmap outlined in this book, movement becomes a critical driver of metabolic restoration, long-term blood sugar stability, and sustainable diabetes reversal.

6. Stress Management

Stress is one of the most powerful yet underestimated drivers of insulin resistance and poor blood sugar control. Both acute and chronic stress can significantly disrupt glucose metabolism, elevate insulin levels, and accelerate the progression of diabetes. Research consistently demonstrates that individuals experiencing chronic psychological stress are at substantially higher risk for insulin resistance, metabolic syndrome, and type 2 diabetes (Hackett & Steptoe, 2017).

Stress does not merely affect emotions. It produces measurable biochemical changes that interfere with insulin signaling, promote inflammation, disrupt sleep, and increase glucose production by the liver. For many individuals, stress is the hidden factor preventing blood sugar improvement despite dietary changes, exercise, and medication adherence.

Physiological Mechanisms Linking Stress to Diabetes

The relationship between stress and diabetes is mediated primarily through activation of the hypothalamic pituitary adrenal axis and the sympathetic nervous system. When the body perceives stress, it releases cortisol, adrenaline, and norepinephrine. These hormones increase blood glucose availability to prepare the body for a perceived threat. Cortisol directly raises blood sugar by stimulating gluconeogenesis in the liver and reducing insulin sensitivity in muscle and adipose tissue (Chrousos, 2009). Chronic elevation of cortisol leads to persistent hyperglycemia, increased visceral fat storage, and worsening insulin resistance. Over time, this hormonal environment contributes to beta cell exhaustion and impaired glucose regulation. A longitudinal study published in *Diabetes Care* found that individuals with high perceived stress had significantly higher fasting glucose levels and increased risk of developing type 2 diabetes independent of body mass index and lifestyle factors (Harris et al., 2017).

Chronic Stress and Insulin Resistance

Unlike short-term stress, which the body can recover from, chronic stress keeps the nervous system in a constant state of activation. This sustained stress response promotes inflammation, oxidative damage, and hormonal imbalance. Elevated cortisol interferes with insulin receptor signaling and promotes central fat accumulation, particularly in the abdominal region. Visceral fat itself produces inflammatory cytokines that further worsen insulin resistance. A meta-analysis by Kyrou et al. (2018) confirmed that chronic psychosocial stress significantly increases insulin resistance and metabolic dysfunction. Stress also impairs sleep quality, disrupts appetite regulation, and increases cravings for refined carbohydrates and sugar, compounding glycemic instability.

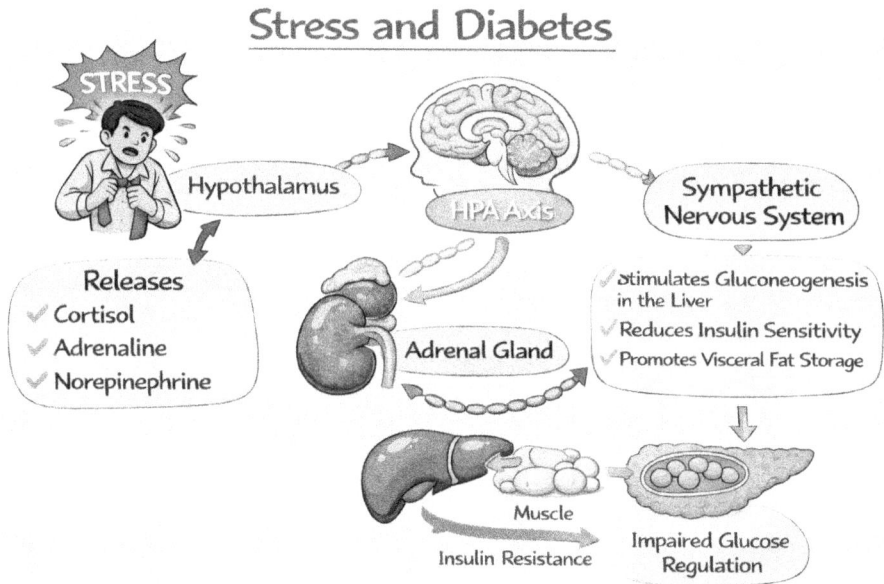

Stress and Diabetes

Stress, Trauma, Anxiety, and Diabetes

Unresolved emotional stress, trauma, anxiety, and depression play a significant role in diabetes development and progression. Individuals with post-traumatic stress disorder and chronic anxiety demonstrate higher fasting glucose levels, increased insulin resistance, and poorer glycemic control compared to non-affected populations (Roberts et al., 2015). Depression is particularly impactful. It alters brain chemistry, increases inflammatory markers, and dysregulates cortisol secretion. Depression is also associated with reduced motivation, poor dietary adherence, disrupted sleep, and decreased physical activity, all of which worsen diabetes outcomes (Mezuk et al., 2008). For individuals experiencing persistent anxiety, depression, or trauma-related stress, addressing emotional health is not optional. It is foundational to metabolic healing.

Effects of Stress on Key Biological Systems

Chronic stress affects nearly every system involved in glucose regulation:

- **Metabolic effects:** Increased blood glucose, insulin resistance, and visceral fat accumulation
- **Cardiovascular effects:** Elevated blood pressure, endothelial dysfunction, and increased cardiovascular risk
- **Neurological effects:** Anxiety, depression, cognitive impairment, and sleep disruption
- **Immune effects:** Increased inflammation and impaired immune regulation
- **Musculoskeletal effects:** Chronic muscle tension, pain, and fatigue
- **Gastrointestinal effects:** Altered gut motility and microbiome imbalance

These overlapping effects explain why unmanaged stress often undermines even the best diabetes treatment plans.

Practical Strategies for Managing Stress

Stress management does not require perfection. It requires consistency. The following evidence-based strategies can significantly improve nervous system regulation and blood sugar control.

Breathing Meditation

Slow, controlled breathing activates the parasympathetic nervous system and reduces cortisol output. A randomized controlled trial demonstrated that diaphragmatic breathing significantly reduced cortisol levels and improved insulin sensitivity in individuals with metabolic dysfunction (Ma et al., 2017).

Simple Practice

Sit comfortably. Inhale through the nose for four seconds, allowing the belly to expand. Exhale slowly through the mouth for six seconds. Repeat for five minutes.

The 4-7-8 Relaxation Breath

This technique reduces sympathetic nervous system activation and improves sleep quality. Inhale for four seconds, hold for seven seconds, exhale for eight seconds. Repeat four times. This method is especially effective before bed or during acute stress.

Mindful Walking

Mindful walking combines gentle movement with nervous system regulation. Studies show that mindful movement reduces stress hormones and improves glucose control more effectively than sedentary relaxation alone (Pascoe et al., 2017). Focus attention on the sensation of your feet, breath, and surroundings for ten to twenty minutes.

Body Scan Meditation

This technique releases stored muscle tension and reduces physiological stress. A study published in *Psychoneuroendocrinology* found that body scan meditation significantly reduced cortisol levels and inflammatory markers (Creswell et al., 2012).

Making Stress Management a Daily Habit

Consistency matters more than duration. Five to ten minutes daily can produce meaningful physiological change. Pair stress reduction with daily routines such as waking, meals, or bedtime. Use reminders. Be patient. Nervous system healing is cumulative.

When Stress Is More Than Lifestyle

While this chapter provides practical tools for everyday stress regulation, it is important to recognize when stress is rooted in deeper anxiety, depression, or unresolved trauma. These conditions require a more comprehensive and structured approach. For readers seeking deeper emotional healing, I strongly recommend my book **Beating Anxiety and Depression**, which provides a research-backed, natural framework for addressing the biological, nutritional, psychological, and lifestyle drivers of anxiety and depression. Restoring emotional balance allows the body to regulate cortisol, insulin, and glucose more effectively, making diabetes reversal far more attainable.

Conclusion: How Stress Management Fits Into the 10 Natural Secrets

Stress management is not an optional add-on in diabetes reversal. It is a core pillar. Chronic stress directly interferes with insulin signaling, raises blood sugar, disrupts sleep, and undermines every other intervention in this book. When stress is regulated, the body becomes more responsive to dietary changes, fasting strategies, nutrient repletion, exercise, medication adjustments, and behavioral change. Stress management enhances the effectiveness of all other natural secrets by restoring hormonal balance and nervous system stability. Diabetes is a complex condition that requires an integrated approach. Addressing stress alongside the other nine natural secrets creates the internal environment necessary for lasting metabolic healing. When the nervous system shifts out of survival mode, the body can finally begin to repair, restore, and rebalance.

BEATING
ANXIETY
&
DEPRESSION

BONUS VIDEOS

14 NATURAL SECRETS TO A HAPPIER LIFE

- Conquer Anxiety & Depression Naturally
- Heal the Root Causes & Reclaim Your Life
- Created by a Doctor Who Conquered PTSD & Depression
- Science-Based Strategies for Lasting Change

Dr. Joseph Jacobs, DPT, ACN

Spine text: BEATING ANXIETY & DEPRESSION · 14 NATURAL SECRETS · JACOBS

7. Environmental Toxins

Environmental toxins are an often overlooked but powerful contributor to insulin resistance and diabetes. Modern life exposes individuals to thousands of chemicals daily through food, water, air, household products, personal care items, medications, and environmental pollution. Many of these compounds interfere directly with glucose metabolism, hormone signaling, mitochondrial function, and pancreatic health. Research increasingly identifies environmental toxins as endocrine-disrupting chemicals, substances that interfere with hormone action even at low doses. Because insulin is a hormone, disruption of endocrine signaling has direct consequences for blood sugar regulation. For many individuals, toxin exposure is a hidden barrier preventing metabolic recovery despite disciplined efforts with diet, exercise, and medications.

How Environmental Toxins Disrupt Glucose Metabolism

Environmental toxins contribute to diabetes through several interconnected mechanisms. Many toxins impair insulin receptor signaling, reduce glucose uptake by muscle cells, and increase oxidative stress. Others directly damage pancreatic beta cells, reducing insulin production. A growing body of evidence demonstrates that exposure to endocrine-disrupting chemicals increases insulin resistance, promotes visceral fat accumulation, and elevates fasting blood glucose levels (Gore et al., 2015). These compounds alter gene expression, disrupt mitochondrial energy production, and create chronic low-grade inflammation that worsens metabolic dysfunction.

Endocrine-Disrupting Chemicals and Diabetes

Endocrine-disrupting chemicals include substances such as bisphenol A, phthalates, pesticides, herbicides, flame retardants, and certain heavy metals. These chemicals mimic or block natural hormones, interfere with insulin signaling, and disrupt glucose homeostasis. A systematic review published in *The Lancet Diabetes and Endocrinology* concluded that endocrine-disrupting chemicals significantly contribute to insulin resistance and the global diabetes burden (Heindel et al., 2017). These effects are particularly concerning because they occur at exposure levels previously considered safe.

Plastics and Chemical Food Packaging

Bisphenol A and related compounds are commonly found in plastic food containers, water bottles, can linings, and thermal receipts. These chemicals leach into food and beverages, especially when heated. Multiple studies have demonstrated that BPA exposure is associated with increased insulin resistance and higher risk of type 2 diabetes (Lang et al., 2008). BPA disrupts pancreatic beta cell function and alters adipocyte metabolism, promoting glucose dysregulation. Phthalates, another class of plasticizers, are linked to impaired insulin sensitivity and increased abdominal fat accumulation. Reducing plastic food contact is a critical step in lowering toxin burden.

Pesticides and Herbicides

Agricultural chemicals such as organophosphates and glyphosate have been shown to interfere with mitochondrial function and insulin signaling. Chronic exposure occurs through non-organic produce, contaminated water, and environmental drift. Epidemiological studies have found higher diabetes prevalence among individuals with occupational pesticide exposure (Montgomery et al., 2008). Glyphosate exposure has also been associated with gut microbiome disruption, which plays a critical role in glucose metabolism.

Heavy Metals

Heavy metals such as mercury, cadmium, arsenic, and lead are toxic to metabolic tissues. These metals accumulate in the body over time and disrupt insulin signaling pathways. Arsenic exposure, even at low levels, has been strongly linked to increased diabetes risk. A review published in *Current Diabetes Reports* confirmed that arsenic impairs insulin secretion and increases insulin resistance (Kuo et al., 2013). Heavy metals also increase oxidative stress and mitochondrial dysfunction, further impairing glucose regulation.

Air Pollution and Metabolic Dysfunction

Airborne pollutants such as particulate matter and nitrogen dioxide contribute to systemic inflammation and insulin resistance. Long-term exposure to air pollution has been associated with increased incidence of type 2 diabetes. A large cohort study found that individuals living in areas with higher air pollution levels had significantly higher fasting glucose and insulin resistance, independent of lifestyle factors (Brook et al., 2013).

Household and Personal Care Products

Many household cleaners, fragrances, cosmetics, and personal care products contain hormone-disrupting chemicals such as parabens and synthetic fragrances. These compounds are absorbed through the skin and respiratory system. Research indicates that exposure to these chemicals contributes to metabolic disruption and increased diabetes risk (Trasande et al., 2013). Fragrance-free and non-toxic alternatives can significantly reduce daily exposure.

The Liver, Detoxification, and Diabetes

The liver plays a central role in both detoxification and glucose regulation. When toxin exposure overwhelms liver detoxification pathways, glucose metabolism becomes impaired. Toxin-induced liver stress increases insulin resistance, promotes fatty liver disease, and worsens glycemic control. Supporting liver function through toxin reduction and nutrient repletion enhances metabolic resilience.

Practical Strategies to Reduce Toxin Exposure

Reducing toxin exposure does not require perfection. Small, consistent changes create meaningful improvements.
• Choose organic produce when possible, especially for high-residue foods
• Avoid heating food in plastic containers
• Use glass or stainless steel food storage
• Filter drinking water
• Choose fragrance-free and non-toxic personal care products
• Reduce consumption of processed foods
• Improve indoor air quality through ventilation and air filtration

These steps reduce cumulative toxin burden and support metabolic healing.

Why Detox Supplements Are Not the Solution

Many products marketed as detox solutions lack scientific support and may strain the liver or kidneys. True detoxification occurs through the liver, kidneys, gut, lungs, and skin, not through aggressive supplementation. Supporting detox pathways requires reducing exposure, correcting nutrient deficiencies, optimizing gut health, and addressing stress and sleep. Supplementation should only be used when clinically indicated and guided by laboratory testing.

Conclusion: How Environmental Toxins Fit Into the 10 Natural Secrets

Environmental toxins represent a hidden but significant contributor to insulin resistance and diabetes progression. Reducing toxin exposure removes a major obstacle to healing and allows the other natural secrets in this book to work more effectively. When toxin burden is lowered, insulin sensitivity improves and systemic inflammation decreases. This allows the body to respond more effectively to nutrition, fasting, exercise, stress management, sleep optimization, nutrient repletion, medication adjustments, and behavioral change. Diabetes is a complex condition driven by multiple interacting factors. Addressing environmental toxins alongside the other nine natural secrets creates a metabolic environment where true healing becomes possible. Reducing exposure is not about fear. It is about empowerment, awareness, and supporting the body's natural ability to restore balance.

8. Sleep

Sleep is one of the most powerful regulators of blood sugar and insulin sensitivity, yet it is one of the most commonly neglected aspects of metabolic health. Chronic sleep deprivation and poor sleep quality significantly increase the risk of insulin resistance, type 2 diabetes, weight gain, and cardiovascular disease. Even modest disruptions in sleep can produce measurable changes in glucose metabolism within days. Research consistently shows that individuals who sleep fewer than six hours per night have a significantly higher risk of developing diabetes compared to those who sleep seven to eight hours consistently (Cappuccio et al., 2010). Sleep is not merely a passive state of rest. It is an active, restorative process during which the body regulates hormones, repairs tissues, stabilizes glucose metabolism, and resets the nervous system.

How Sleep Regulates Blood Sugar

Sleep plays a central role in glucose regulation through its effects on insulin sensitivity, cortisol balance, appetite hormones, and autonomic nervous system activity. During deep sleep, insulin sensitivity improves, inflammation decreases, and glucose utilization becomes more efficient. Sleep deprivation disrupts this balance. Studies demonstrate that even one night of partial sleep loss reduces insulin sensitivity by up to 25 percent (Spiegel et al., 1999). Chronic sleep restriction leads to sustained elevations in fasting glucose, increased insulin resistance, and impaired pancreatic beta cell function.

Cortisol, Sleep, and Insulin Resistance

Sleep deprivation causes dysregulation of the hypothalamic pituitary adrenal axis, leading to elevated evening and nighttime cortisol levels. Cortisol directly raises blood glucose by stimulating hepatic gluconeogenesis and inhibiting insulin action in peripheral tissues. A controlled laboratory study published in *The Journal of Clinical Endocrinology and Metabolism* found that individuals exposed to sleep restriction had significantly higher evening cortisol levels and impaired glucose tolerance (Leproult & Van Cauter, 2010). Over time, this hormonal pattern contributes to persistent hyperglycemia and worsening insulin resistance.

Sleep and Appetite Hormones

Sleep has a profound effect on appetite regulation through its influence on leptin and ghrelin. Leptin signals satiety, while ghrelin stimulates hunger. Inadequate sleep lowers leptin levels and raises ghrelin levels, increasing hunger and cravings, particularly for refined carbohydrates and sugar. A landmark study demonstrated that sleep restriction resulted in a 24 percent increase in hunger and a strong preference for high-glycemic foods (Spiegel et al., 2004). This hormonal imbalance makes dietary adherence significantly more difficult and accelerates blood sugar instability.

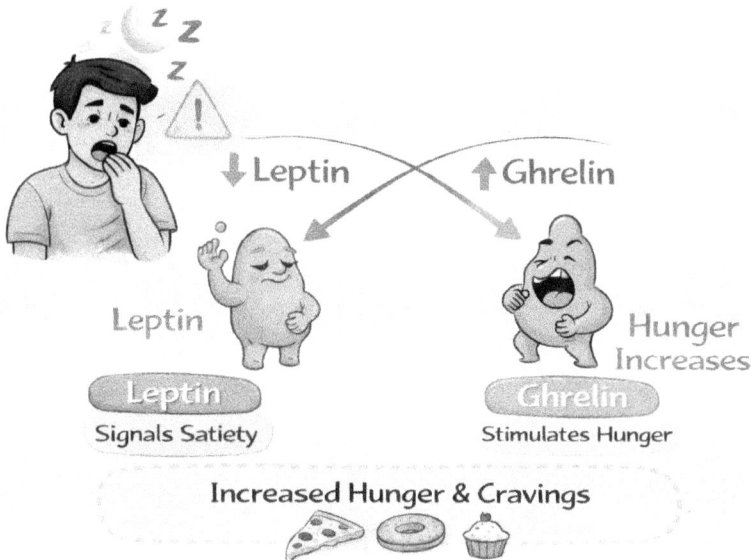

Lack of Sleep and Appetite Hormones

↓Leptin ↑Ghrelin

Leptin Hunger Increases

Leptin — Signals Satiety

Ghrelin — Stimulates Hunger

Increased Hunger & Cravings

Sleep Apnea and Diabetes

Obstructive sleep apnea is highly prevalent in individuals with insulin resistance and type 2 diabetes. Repeated episodes of oxygen deprivation during sleep activate stress pathways, increase inflammation, and worsen insulin resistance. A meta-analysis published in *Diabetes Care* confirmed that untreated sleep apnea is independently associated with poor glycemic control and increased diabetes risk (Reutrakul & Van Cauter, 2018). Addressing sleep-disordered breathing is essential for individuals with resistant or poorly controlled diabetes.

Circadian Rhythm Disruption

The body's internal clock regulates insulin secretion, glucose uptake, and hormone release. Disruptions in circadian rhythm, such as shift work, irregular sleep schedules, and late-night screen exposure, impair glucose metabolism. A prospective study of shift workers found significantly higher rates of insulin resistance and type 2 diabetes compared to day workers (Gan et al., 2015). Consistency in sleep timing is just as important as sleep duration for metabolic health.

Stress, Sleep, and Blood Sugar

Stress and sleep are deeply interconnected. Poor sleep increases stress hormone output, while chronic stress disrupts sleep architecture. This bidirectional relationship amplifies insulin resistance and glucose instability. Individuals with chronic anxiety or depression frequently experience sleep fragmentation, early awakenings, or difficulty falling asleep. Addressing emotional stress, as discussed in earlier chapters, is often necessary to restore healthy sleep patterns and improve glycemic control.

Practical Strategies to Improve Sleep Quality

Improving sleep does not require perfection. Small, consistent changes can significantly improve metabolic outcomes.

- **Establish a Consistent Sleep Schedule:** Go to bed and wake up at the same time daily, including weekends. Consistency strengthens circadian rhythm regulation.
- **Reduce Evening Light Exposure:** Blue light from screens suppresses melatonin production. Avoid screens at least one hour before bedtime or use blue light filters.
- **Create a Sleep-Supportive Environment:** Keep the bedroom cool, dark, and quiet. Darkness signals melatonin release and promotes deeper sleep stages.
- **Avoid Late-Night Eating:** Eating late elevates insulin and disrupts nocturnal glucose regulation. Aim to finish meals at least four to five hours before bedtime.

- **Limit Stimulants:** Caffeine and other stimulants can impair sleep quality even when consumed earlier in the day. Sensitivity varies, and individualized limits may be necessary.
- **Support Relaxation Before Bed:** Gentle stretching, breathing exercises, prayer, or mindfulness practices help shift the nervous system into a parasympathetic state.

Why Sleep Medications Are Not the Solution

While sleep medications may offer short-term relief, they do not restore natural sleep architecture and may worsen insulin resistance over time. Many sedatives suppress deep sleep stages critical for glucose regulation. Long-term reliance on sleep medications has been associated with metabolic disruption, cognitive impairment, and increased fall risk. Addressing the root causes of poor sleep, such as stress, circadian misalignment, nutrient deficiencies, or sleep apnea, is a safer and more effective approach.

Conclusion: How Sleep Fits Into the 10 Natural Secrets

Sleep is a foundational pillar of diabetes reversal. Without adequate, restorative sleep, insulin sensitivity declines, cortisol rises, appetite regulation fails, and blood sugar control becomes increasingly difficult. Improving sleep enhances the effectiveness of every other natural secret in this book. When sleep is restored, the body becomes more responsive to nutrition, fasting, exercise, stress management, toxin reduction, nutrient repletion, medication adjustments, and behavioral change. Diabetes is a complex condition that requires a comprehensive approach. Addressing sleep alongside the other nine natural secrets creates the hormonal and neurological environment necessary for lasting metabolic healing. When the body is well rested, it is far more capable of repairing, rebalancing, and restoring healthy glucose regulation.

9. Fasting

9. Fasting

Fasting is one of the most effective tools for improving insulin sensitivity and restoring metabolic flexibility when implemented correctly. Unlike calorie restriction alone, fasting works by lowering circulating insulin levels, allowing the body to shift from constant glucose dependence toward fat utilization and cellular repair. When practiced improperly, however, fasting can worsen blood sugar instability, increase stress hormones, and undermine metabolic health. For this reason, fasting must always be paired with **nutrient-dense eating, appropriate meal timing, and individualized guidance**.

Fasting is a foundational component of the **ASTR Diet**, a comprehensive nutritional framework detailed in *Eat to Heal*. Within this approach, fasting is not about deprivation. It is a strategic period of metabolic rest that supports insulin regulation, inflammation reduction, and tissue repair, while daytime meals are intentionally designed to nourish the body and stabilize blood sugar.

How Fasting Improves Insulin Sensitivity

Insulin resistance develops when insulin remains elevated for prolonged periods, often due to frequent eating, refined carbohydrates, and chronic stress. Fasting lowers basal insulin levels and improves insulin receptor responsiveness, allowing glucose to be cleared from the bloodstream more efficiently. Clinical studies demonstrate that intermittent fasting improves insulin sensitivity, reduces fasting glucose, and lowers HbA1c in individuals with insulin resistance and type 2 diabetes (Patterson et al., 2015). By reducing the frequency of insulin spikes, fasting gives pancreatic beta cells an opportunity to recover and reduces metabolic strain.

Fasting, Glucose Regulation, and Metabolic Flexibility

Metabolic flexibility refers to the body's ability to switch efficiently between glucose and fat as fuel sources. In insulin-resistant states, this flexibility is impaired. Fasting restores metabolic flexibility by promoting lipolysis and increasing reliance on fatty acids and ketones for energy. A randomized controlled trial found that time-restricted eating improved insulin sensitivity and reduced oxidative stress independent of weight loss (Sutton et al., 2018). These benefits are particularly relevant for individuals who struggle with post-meal glucose spikes and persistent hyperinsulinemia.

Fasting and Cellular Repair

One of fasting's most powerful benefits is its role in activating autophagy, a cellular cleanup process that removes damaged proteins and organelles. Autophagy improves mitochondrial efficiency, reduces inflammation, and supports insulin signaling. Animal and human studies show that fasting-induced autophagy improves metabolic health and reduces markers of insulin resistance (de Cabo & Mattson, 2019). This process cannot occur effectively when insulin levels remain chronically elevated, which is common with frequent eating patterns.

Why Fasting Must Be Combined With Healthy Eating

Fasting alone is not enough. Breaking a fast with inflammatory foods, refined carbohydrates, or excessive sugar negates many of fasting's metabolic benefits and may worsen glucose instability. The **ASTR Diet** emphasizes that fasting must be paired with **anti-inflammatory, toxin-free, restorative meals** during eating windows. Nutrient-dense meals stabilize blood sugar, reduce cortisol output, and prevent rebound hyperglycemia. Protein, healthy fats, fiber-rich carbohydrates, and micronutrient sufficiency are essential for fasting to be safe and effective. Research confirms that fasting combined with high-quality nutrition produces superior metabolic outcomes compared to fasting paired with poor dietary quality (Anton et al., 2018).

Meal Timing and Circadian Alignment

The timing of meals plays a critical role in fasting effectiveness. Eating earlier in the day aligns food intake with circadian insulin sensitivity, which is highest in the morning and early afternoon. A controlled feeding study demonstrated that early time-restricted eating significantly improved insulin sensitivity and reduced fasting insulin compared to later eating windows (Sutton et al., 2018). Late-night eating disrupts circadian rhythm, elevates insulin overnight, and impairs glucose regulation. The ASTR Diet prioritizes **daytime eating windows** and **overnight fasting** to support circadian biology and metabolic health.

Who Should Use Caution With Fasting

Fasting is not appropriate for everyone without modification. Individuals with advanced diabetes, a history of eating disorders, adrenal dysfunction, pregnancy, or those taking insulin or glucose-lowering medications require professional supervision. Unsupervised fasting may lead to hypoglycemia, dizziness, fatigue, hormonal dysregulation, or increased cortisol output. For this reason, fasting protocols must be **individualized and adjusted** based on metabolic status, lifestyle, and medication use.

Common Fasting Mistakes
Several mistakes can undermine fasting benefits:

• Skipping meals while consuming poor-quality foods
• Fasting for prolonged periods without nutrient repletion
• Combining fasting with excessive caffeine or stimulants
• Ignoring sleep, stress, and hydration
• Applying rigid protocols without personalization

Fasting should support healing, not create additional stress on the body.

Practical Fasting Guidelines Within the ASTR Diet

Within the ASTR framework, fasting is implemented gradually and intentionally:

• Begin with an overnight fast of 12 hours
• Progress to 14 to 16 hours only if well tolerated
• Consume nutrient-dense meals during eating windows
• Avoid late-night eating
• Monitor energy, mood, and blood sugar response

Because fasting interacts with many physiological systems, **it is difficult to fully explain its implementation in a single chapter**. For complete guidance on how to apply fasting safely and effectively, including personalized strategies, meal composition, and timing, refer to *Eat to Heal*, which provides a step-by-step approach to fasting within the ASTR Diet.

Conclusion: How Fasting Fits Into the 10 Natural Secrets

Fasting is a powerful metabolic tool when used correctly, but it is not a standalone solution. Its effectiveness depends on what you eat, when you eat, how you manage stress, how you sleep, and how well nutrient deficiencies and medication effects are addressed. Within the ASTR Diet, fasting works synergistically with nutrient-dense eating, stress regulation, sleep optimization, toxin reduction, exercise, and behavioral change. When fasting is integrated thoughtfully with the other natural secrets in this book, insulin sensitivity improves, inflammation decreases, and metabolic balance becomes attainable. Diabetes is a complex condition that requires precision and integration. Fasting, when combined with proper nutrition and timing, supports the body's natural ability to heal. For those seeking a complete, structured roadmap for implementing fasting safely and effectively, *Eat to Heal* provides the comprehensive guidance needed to make fasting a sustainable and restorative part of long-term metabolic health.

10. Behavior Modification

Behavioral modification plays a foundational role in reversing diabetes. Unlike medications that focus primarily on controlling blood sugar numbers, behavior change addresses the root drivers of insulin resistance and metabolic dysfunction. Diabetes does not develop overnight, and it cannot be reversed with isolated actions or short-term efforts. Sustainable healing occurs when daily habits are intentionally reshaped to support the body's natural ability to regulate blood glucose, repair insulin signaling, and reduce chronic inflammation. The ten natural secrets presented throughout this book are not independent strategies. Each one contributes to the development or reversal of diabetes. Behavioral modification is the mechanism that allows these principles to work together as an integrated lifestyle rather than as disconnected interventions.

Why Behavioral Change Is Essential in Diabetes Reversal

Diabetes is a complex metabolic condition influenced by food choices, stress, sleep, physical activity, medications, nutrient status, environmental exposures, and emotional patterns. When unhealthy behaviors are repeated daily, the body adapts by becoming insulin resistant. When supportive behaviors are practiced consistently, the body adapts by restoring metabolic flexibility. Behavior change is not about discipline or perfection. It is about creating structure, awareness, and consistency. The goal is to make health-supportive behaviors automatic and sustainable so that blood sugar control becomes a natural outcome rather than a constant struggle.

Core Behavioral Modification Strategies for Reversing Diabetes

1. Dietary Behavior Change

Food choices are one of the most powerful drivers of insulin resistance or insulin sensitivity. Following the ASTR Diet provides a structured, evidence-based approach to changing dietary behaviors in a way that supports metabolic healing. Detailed in *Eat to Heal*, the ASTR Diet focuses on anti-inflammatory, sustainable, toxin-free, and restorative nutrition. Behavioral change in this area means moving away from reactive eating, emotional eating, and convenience-based food decisions. It involves intentional meal timing, nutrient-dense food selection, and consistency. Eliminating refined carbohydrates, added sugars, processed foods, and inflammatory oils while prioritizing whole foods allows insulin sensitivity to improve over time.

2. Consistent Physical Activity

Regular movement improves glucose uptake by muscles, enhances insulin sensitivity, and reduces systemic inflammation. Behavioral modification emphasizes consistency over intensity. Simple strategies such as walking for 30 minutes once or twice daily can significantly improve blood sugar control. For individuals unable to walk due to weather, physical limitations, or scheduling challenges, alternatives such as a desktop exercise bike, resistance bands, or light indoor movement while watching television can be equally effective. The key behavioral shift is removing the "all-or-nothing" mindset and replacing it with daily movement as a non-negotiable habit.

3. Stress Regulation as a Daily Practice

Chronic stress elevates cortisol, disrupts insulin signaling, and contributes to persistent blood sugar elevation. Behavioral change requires making stress regulation part of daily life rather than an occasional response to overwhelm. Practices such as deep breathing, prayer, mindfulness, journaling, and scheduled breaks help regulate the nervous system. When anxiety, depression, or unresolved trauma are present, addressing emotional health becomes essential for metabolic healing. For deeper support, readers are encouraged to explore *Beating Anxiety and Depression* book, which provides a comprehensive, natural framework for emotional and nervous system regulation.

4. Sleep Optimization

Sleep deprivation directly worsens insulin resistance and appetite regulation. Behavioral modification includes setting consistent sleep and wake times, limiting evening screen exposure, and prioritizing 7 to 9 hours of restorative sleep. Poor sleep often undermines even the best nutrition and exercise efforts. Making sleep a priority rather than an afterthought is a critical behavior shift for diabetes reversal.

5. Reducing Harmful Exposures

Environmental toxins, ultra-processed foods, endocrine disruptors, and unnecessary medications can all worsen insulin resistance. Behavioral change involves increasing awareness and making gradual, intentional choices to reduce exposure. This includes reading labels, simplifying household products, choosing cleaner food sources, and working with healthcare providers to review medications that may impair metabolic health.

6. Accountability and Professional Support

Behavior change is far more effective with guidance and accountability. Working with an advanced clinical nutritionist and a healthcare provider trained in metabolic health provides structure, safety, and personalization. Professional support helps identify blind spots, adjust strategies, interpret lab results, and safely guide changes related to medications, fasting, supplementation, and lifestyle modifications.

7. Tracking Progress Without Obsession

Tracking behaviors such as food intake, movement, sleep patterns, and blood glucose trends can reinforce progress and highlight patterns. Behavioral modification focuses on using data as feedback, not judgment. Setting realistic goals, celebrating small wins, and focusing on trends rather than perfection increases long-term success and reduces burnout.

Behavioral Patterns That Commonly Block Healing

Many individuals struggle to reverse diabetes because of unrecognized behavioral patterns, including:

- Inconsistent eating schedules
- Skipping meals followed by overeating
- Using food to manage stress or emotions
- Exercising sporadically or excessively
- Ignoring sleep quality
- Taking supplements without guidance
- Relying solely on medications without addressing root causes

Replacing these patterns with intentional, repeatable behaviors is essential for lasting metabolic change.

Conclusion

Reversing diabetes requires more than knowledge. It requires daily alignment between behavior and biology. Each chapter in this book addressed a different contributor to insulin resistance. Behavioral modification is what brings these principles to life. When food choices, movement, stress regulation, sleep, nutrient balance, fasting, and environmental awareness are practiced consistently, the body responds. Insulin sensitivity improves, blood sugar stabilizes, and energy increases. Under proper medical supervision, dependence on medications may decrease. This is not about quick fixes; it is about building a lifestyle that supports long-term metabolic health.

Building a Healthier Future

This journey is about more than reversing diabetes. It is about reclaiming vitality, confidence, and freedom. It is about living without constant fear of blood sugar swings, complications, or progressive decline. You are not broken. Your body is adaptive. When given the right signals consistently, it remembers how to heal. Commit to the process. Take small, steady steps. Trust the structure laid out in these ten natural secrets. Healing is not only possible. It is sustainable when behavior aligns with biology.

Conclusion

The Ten Natural Secrets to Reversing Diabetes

Reversing diabetes is not about managing numbers or suppressing symptoms. It is about restoring balance to a system that has been under metabolic stress for years. Diabetes develops when insulin resistance, inflammation, hormonal disruption, and lifestyle stressors accumulate over time. Healing requires addressing each of these contributors together, not in isolation. The ten natural secrets presented in this book form a complete, evidence-supported roadmap. Each one targets a different root cause of diabetes. When implemented together, they create the biological and behavioral conditions necessary for lasting metabolic recovery.

1. Food-Induced Diabetes

Food is one of the most powerful drivers of insulin resistance. Refined carbohydrates, added sugars, ultra-processed foods, inflammatory oils, and hidden food sensitivities repeatedly spike blood sugar and insulin. Over time, this leads to chronic hyperinsulinemia and impaired glucose regulation. Healing begins by removing inflammatory foods and adopting a whole-food, anti-inflammatory eating pattern that stabilizes blood sugar and restores insulin sensitivity. Consistency matters more than perfection. When food becomes a therapeutic tool rather than a metabolic stressor, the body can begin to heal.

2. Drug-Induced Diabetes

Many commonly prescribed medications worsen insulin resistance and elevate blood sugar. Corticosteroids, antidepressants, statins, beta blockers, and certain blood pressure medications can silently undermine metabolic health. Reversing diabetes requires reviewing medications with a qualified healthcare provider and safely reducing, replacing, or eliminating drugs that impair insulin sensitivity whenever possible. This process must be done carefully and under medical supervision. Medications should support healing, not interfere with it.

3. Medicinal Teas

Medicinal teas offer gentle yet meaningful metabolic support when used consistently. Teas such as green tea, hibiscus, cinnamon, rooibos, chamomile, and ginger contain plant compounds that reduce inflammation, improve insulin sensitivity, and support nervous system regulation. Incorporating medicinal teas into daily routines provides a simple, calming ritual that reinforces healing throughout the day. Small habits, repeated consistently, produce powerful effects over time.

4. Vitamin, Mineral, and Hormonal Imbalances

Most individuals with diabetes have multiple nutrient deficiencies that impair insulin signaling and glucose metabolism. Common deficiencies include magnesium, vitamin D, B vitamins, zinc, potassium, and iron. Hormonal imbalances involving cortisol, thyroid hormones, and sex hormones further worsen insulin resistance. Correcting these imbalances requires lab-guided testing and personalized intervention. Supplementing without proper guidance can be ineffective or harmful. Working with an clinical nutritionist ensures proper assessment, correct dosing, and safe implementation.

5. Stress Management

Chronic stress elevates cortisol, disrupts insulin signaling, increases inflammation, and drives persistent blood sugar elevation. Stress management is not optional in diabetes reversal. Daily practices such as deep breathing, mindfulness, prayer, journaling, and nervous system regulation help shift the body out of survival mode and into a state of repair. Addressing anxiety, depression, and unresolved trauma is essential for long-term metabolic stability. For readers who are navigating anxiety, depression, or past trauma, additional guidance is available in *Beating Anxiety and Depression*. That book explores natural, science-informed strategies for supporting mental health through nutrition, nervous system regulation, cognitive reframing, behavioral change, and restorative habits. Addressing emotional health alongside metabolic health creates the conditions needed for lasting blood sugar stability and whole-body healing.

6. Environmental Toxins

Endocrine-disrupting chemicals found in plastics, pesticides, household cleaners, cosmetics, and processed foods interfere with insulin signaling and hormone regulation. Chronic toxin exposure places additional strain on metabolic systems already under stress. Reducing toxic burden through cleaner food choices, safer household products, and simplified personal care routines lowers physiological stress and supports insulin sensitivity.

7. Sleep

Poor sleep alone can drive insulin resistance, increase cravings, and destabilize blood sugar. Sleep deprivation disrupts cortisol rhythms, appetite hormones, and glucose metabolism. Consistently getting seven to nine hours of restorative sleep helps regulate insulin response and supports metabolic repair. Prioritizing sleep through routine, reduced evening screen exposure, and a supportive sleep environment is essential for diabetes reversal.

8. Fasting

Fasting, when done correctly, improves insulin sensitivity and metabolic flexibility. As part of the ASTR Diet, fasting must be paired with nourishing daytime meals and proper timing. Fasting is not appropriate for everyone, especially individuals with diabetes. It should always be supervised by a clinical nutritionist and healthcare provider trained in metabolic health to prevent hypoglycemia and ensure safety. When applied correctly, fasting becomes a powerful tool rather than a metabolic stressor.

9. Exercise

Regular movement improves glucose uptake, reduces insulin resistance, and lowers inflammation. Exercise does not need to be extreme to be effective. Simple daily walking for thirty minutes once or twice per day significantly improves blood sugar control. For those unable to walk due to weather, injury, or other limitations, alternatives such as desk bikes, light resistance training, or indoor movement while watching television provide meaningful benefits. Consistency matters more than intensity.

10. Behavioral Modification and Integration

Behavioral modification is the foundation that allows all other secrets to work together. Knowledge alone does not reverse diabetes. Healing occurs when daily habits align with biology. Replacing reactive patterns with intentional routines around food, movement, sleep, stress, and environment allows the body to restore metabolic balance. Sustainable change happens when healthy behaviors become automatic rather than forced.

Conclusion: A New Way Forward

Reversing diabetes is not about fighting your body. It is about learning how to work with it again. Diabetes does not develop from a single mistake, and it cannot be reversed with a single solution. It emerges from the interaction of biological imbalance, chronic stress, and repeated lifestyle patterns. That same complexity is what makes healing possible. When those contributors are addressed together, the body responds. The ten natural secrets in this book form a complete, integrated roadmap. Each one addresses a different driver of insulin resistance. When implemented together, they reduce metabolic stress, restore insulin sensitivity, and create the conditions needed for lasting healing. This journey is not about perfection. It is about progress. Small, steady changes practiced consistently are far more powerful than extreme efforts that cannot be sustained. Even modest improvements, repeated daily, can shift metabolism in a meaningful way over time.

You are not broken. Your body is adaptive, resilient, and designed to respond to the signals it receives most often. When you provide nourishment instead of stress, rest instead of exhaustion, movement instead of stagnation, and calm instead of constant pressure, your biology responds. Let this book be a guide, not a burden. Apply what you have learned at a pace that feels realistic and sustainable. Seek professional support when needed. Partner with practitioners who understand metabolic health and can guide you safely. Healing is not only possible. It is attainable, sustainable, and within reach. The roadmap is now in your hands. The next step is simply to begin.

Recommended Resources

How to Access Online Content
1. Open the camera app on your smartphone.
2. Point the camera at the barcode.
3. A notification will appear with a link. Tap the notification to open the link in your browser.

Limited Time Offer: FREE 30-minute Health Coach Consultation

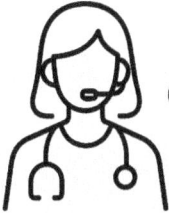

FREE
CONSULTATION
WITH
HEALTH COACH

GET STARTED

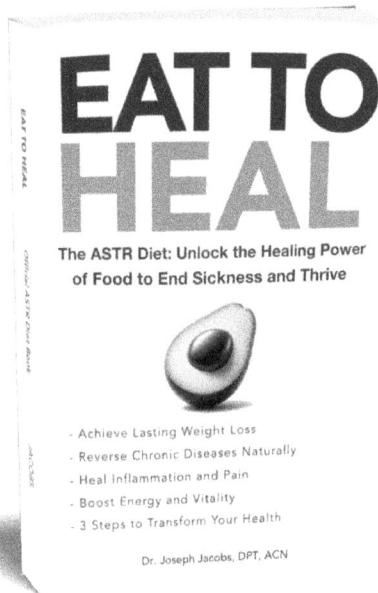

EAT TO HEAL

The ASTR Diet: Unlock the Healing Power of Food to End Sickness and Thrive

- Achieve Lasting Weight Loss
- Reverse Chronic Diseases Naturally
- Heal Inflammation and Pain
- Boost Energy and Vitality
- 3 Steps to Transform Your Health

Dr. Joseph Jacobs, DPT, ACN

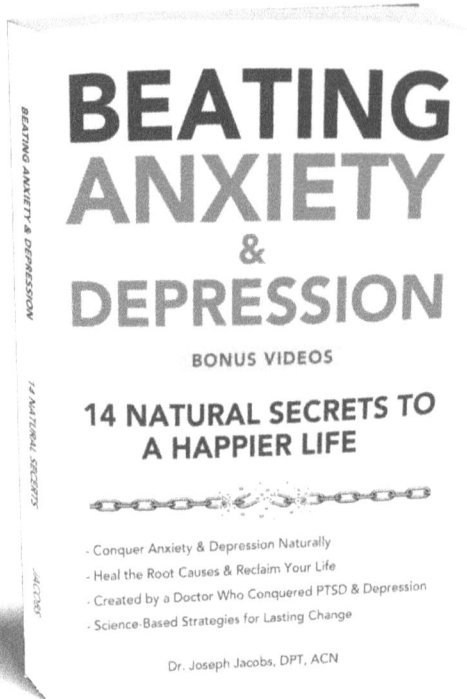

BEATING
ANXIETY
&
DEPRESSION

BONUS VIDEOS

14 NATURAL SECRETS TO
A HAPPIER LIFE

- Conquer Anxiety & Depression Naturally
- Heal the Root Causes & Reclaim Your Life
- Created by a Doctor Who Conquered PTSD & Depression
- Science-Based Strategies for Lasting Change

Dr. Joseph Jacobs, DPT, ACN

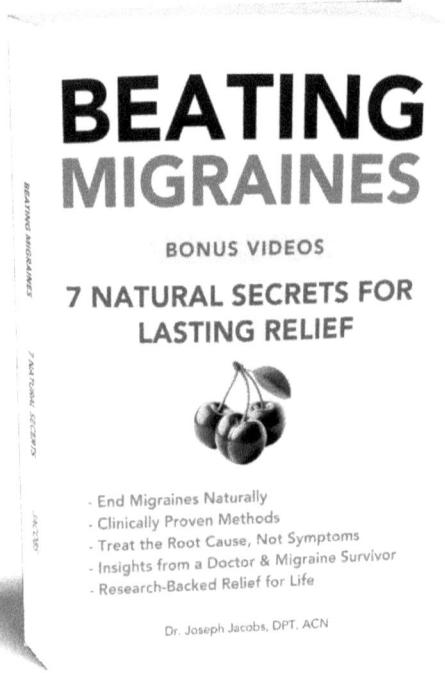

BEATING
MIGRAINES

BONUS VIDEOS

7 NATURAL SECRETS FOR
LASTING RELIEF

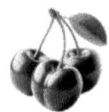

- End Migraines Naturally
- Clinically Proven Methods
- Treat the Root Cause, Not Symptoms
- Insights from a Doctor & Migraine Survivor
- Research-Backed Relief for Life

Dr. Joseph Jacobs, DPT, ACN

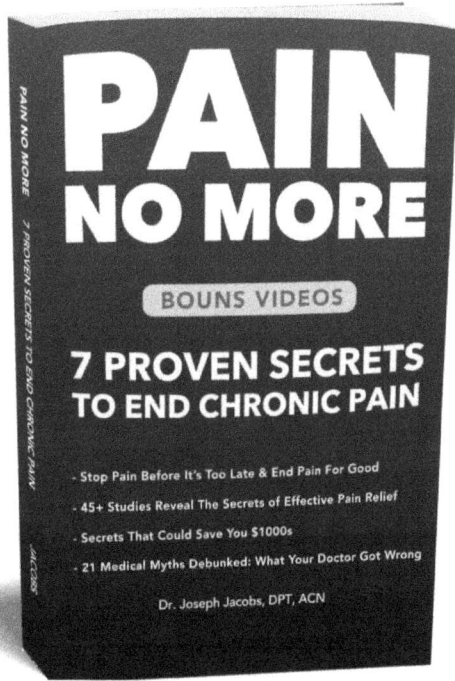

PAIN NO MORE

BOUNS VIDEOS

7 PROVEN SECRETS
TO END CHRONIC PAIN

- Stop Pain Before It's Too Late & End Pain For Good
- 45+ Studies Reveal The Secrets of Effective Pain Relief
- Secrets That Could Save You $1000s
- 21 Medical Myths Debunked: What Your Doctor Got Wrong

Dr. Joseph Jacobs, DPT, ACN

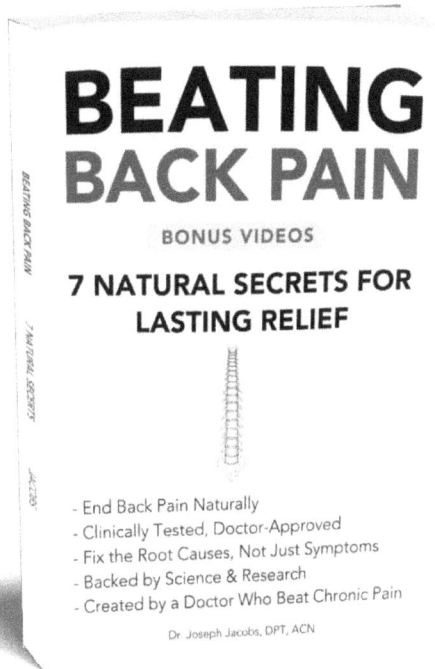

BEATING
BACK PAIN

BONUS VIDEOS

7 NATURAL SECRETS FOR
LASTING RELIEF

- End Back Pain Naturally
- Clinically Tested, Doctor-Approved
- Fix the Root Causes, Not Just Symptoms
- Backed by Science & Research
- Created by a Doctor Who Beat Chronic Pain

Dr. Joseph Jacobs, DPT, ACN

REVERSING
HIGH BLOOD
PRESSURE

7 NATURAL SECRETS TO SAFELY
LOWER BLOOD PRESSURE

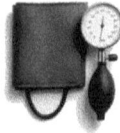

- Natural Solutions That Work
- Backed by Extensive Research
- Fix the Root Cause, Not Just the Numbers
- No Drugs, No Side Effects

Dr. Joseph Jacobs, DPT, ACN

KILLED BY
FRAGRANCE
How Synthetic Scents Make Us Sick

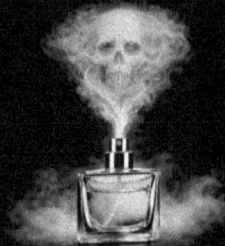

- Exposed by peer-reviewed research
- Links everyday fragrance exposure to chronic disease
- Built on science, not opinion

Dr. Joseph Jacobs, DPT, ACN

Your
SHOES
HURT YOU

Why Does Your Pain Keep Coming
Back and *How to Fix It*

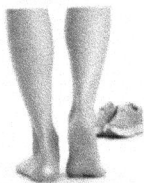

BONUS VIDEOS

- Fix Your Feet. Fix Your Pain.
- Why Modern Shoes Create Chronic Pain
- Backed by Biomechanics and Clinical Research

Dr. Joseph Jacobs, DPT, ACN

Advanced Clinical Nutritionist: A healthcare professional trained to evaluate biochemical, nutritional, and metabolic imbalances using laboratory testing and to design personalized nutrition and supplementation strategies that address root causes of chronic disease rather than symptoms alone.

Alcohol: A metabolic toxin that disrupts liver function, impairs glucose regulation, and worsens insulin resistance. Regular alcohol intake increases the risk of type 2 diabetes and metabolic dysfunction.

Artificial Sweeteners: Non-nutritive compounds such as aspartame, sucralose, and saccharin that replace sugar. Although calorie-free, they may disrupt gut microbiota and impair glucose regulation in some individuals.

ASTR Diet: A comprehensive nutritional framework detailed in *Eat to Heal*. ASTR stands for Anti-inflammatory, Sustainable, Toxin-free, and Restorative, emphasizing whole foods and metabolic balance to address chronic disease at the root.

Behavioral Modification: The process of changing daily habits and routines to support long-term health. In diabetes reversal, this includes consistent practices related to nutrition, movement, sleep, stress regulation, and environmental choices.

Beta Cells: Insulin-producing cells located in the pancreas. Chronic insulin resistance places prolonged stress on beta cells, eventually contributing to dysfunction and type 2 diabetes.

Biopsychosocial Model: A health framework recognizing disease as the result of interacting biological, psychological, and behavioral factors, forming the foundation of the approach used in this book.

Blood Glucose: The amount of glucose present in the bloodstream at any given time, regulated primarily by insulin and influenced by food intake, stress, sleep, and activity.

Chronic Inflammation: A prolonged immune response that interferes with insulin signaling, damages tissues, and contributes to metabolic disease and insulin resistance.

Cortisol: A stress hormone released by the adrenal glands that raises blood sugar, worsens insulin resistance, and promotes fat storage when chronically elevated.

Dehydration: A state of insufficient body fluids that increases stress hormone release and worsens insulin resistance and blood sugar instability.

Glossary

Endocrine Disruptors: Chemicals that interfere with hormone signaling, commonly found in plastics, pesticides, cosmetics, and household cleaners, and linked to insulin resistance and metabolic dysfunction.

Environmental Toxins: Harmful substances found in food, water, air, and consumer products that place stress on the liver, hormones, and metabolic systems.

Fasting: A structured period without caloric intake that, when properly timed and supervised, can improve insulin sensitivity and metabolic flexibility. In this book, fasting is presented as part of the ASTR Diet.

Fasting Insulin: A blood test measuring insulin levels after an overnight fast, used as an early marker of insulin resistance often before blood glucose becomes abnormal.

Food Sensitivity: A delayed immune or inflammatory response to specific foods that may cause fatigue, brain fog, digestive discomfort, joint pain, or blood sugar instability rather than immediate allergic reactions.

Glycemic Load: A measure of how much a food raises blood glucose based on both carbohydrate quality and quantity.

Hyperinsulinemia: A condition characterized by chronically elevated insulin levels that often precedes type 2 diabetes and drives insulin resistance.

Inflammation: The body's immune response to injury or stress that, when chronic, disrupts insulin signaling and contributes to metabolic disease.

Insulin: A hormone produced by the pancreas that allows glucose to enter cells for energy. Insulin resistance occurs when cells respond poorly to insulin.

Insulin Resistance: A condition in which cells become less responsive to insulin, forcing the pancreas to produce more insulin to maintain normal blood sugar levels. This is the primary underlying cause of type 2 diabetes.

Magnesium Deficiency: A common nutritional deficiency associated with impaired insulin signaling and poor glucose control due to magnesium's role in carbohydrate metabolism.

Medicinal Teas: Herbal teas used for therapeutic purposes that contain plant compounds supporting blood sugar regulation, reducing inflammation, and calming the nervous system.

Metabolic Flexibility: The body's ability to efficiently switch between burning glucose and fat for energy, which is impaired in insulin resistance.

Metabolic Syndrome: A cluster of conditions including elevated blood sugar, abdominal obesity, high blood pressure, and abnormal cholesterol levels that significantly increase the risk of type 2 diabetes and cardiovascular disease.

Omega-6 Fatty Acids: Polyunsaturated fats found primarily in industrial seed oils that promote inflammation and worsen insulin resistance when consumed in excess.

Pancreas: An organ responsible for producing insulin and digestive enzymes, which becomes stressed under prolonged insulin resistance.

Prediabetes: A metabolic condition characterized by elevated blood glucose or insulin levels that are not yet in the diabetic range and is often reversible with lifestyle and metabolic intervention.

Processed Foods: Foods altered from their natural state through refining, additives, preservatives, or industrial processing that commonly worsen insulin resistance.

Refined Carbohydrates: Carbohydrates stripped of fiber and nutrients, such as white flour and sugar, that rapidly raise blood glucose and insulin levels.

Stress Response: The body's physiological reaction to perceived threat involving cortisol and adrenaline release, which worsens insulin resistance when chronically activated.

Type 1 Diabetes: An autoimmune condition in which the immune system destroys insulin-producing beta cells of the pancreas, requiring lifelong insulin therapy. It is not caused by lifestyle factors and is not reversible through diet or behavioral changes. This book primarily focuses on prediabetes and type 2 diabetes.

Type 2 Diabetes: A metabolic condition characterized by insulin resistance and impaired glucose regulation that is strongly influenced by lifestyle and environmental factors and is often reversible when root causes are addressed.

Ultra-Processed Foods: Highly manufactured foods containing additives, preservatives, refined sugars, and industrial oils that are strongly associated with insulin resistance and increased diabetes risk.

Vitamin D Deficiency: A common nutritional deficiency linked to impaired insulin secretion, increased inflammation, and higher risk of insulin resistance and type 2 diabetes.

References

1. Röder PV, Wu B, Liu Y, Han W. Pancreatic regulation of glucose homeostasis. Exp Mol Med. 2016;48(3):e219. doi:10.1038/emm.2016.6
2. Rui L. Energy metabolism in the liver. Compr Physiol. 2014;4(1):177-197. doi:10.1002/cphy.c130024
3. American Diabetes Association. Classification and diagnosis of diabetes: Standards of medical care in diabetes—2023. Diabetes Care. 2023;46(Suppl 1):S19-S40. doi:10.2337/dc23-S002
4. Centers for Disease Control and Prevention. Diabetes symptoms. https://www.cdc.gov/diabetes/basics/symptoms.html. Published April 2023. Accessed July 5, 2025.
5. Tabák AG, Herder C, Rathmann W, Brunner EJ, Kivimäki M. Prediabetes: A high-risk state for diabetes development. Lancet. 2012;379(9833):2279-2290. doi:10.1016/S0140-6736(12)60283-9
6. Grundy SM. Metabolic syndrome update. Trends Cardiovasc Med. 2016;26(4):364-373. doi:10.1016/j.tcm.2015.10.004
7. Samson SL, Garber AJ. Metabolic syndrome. Endocrinol Metab Clin North Am. 2014;43(1):1-23. doi:10.1016/j.ecl.2013.09.009
8. Joseph JJ, Golden SH. Cortisol dysregulation: the bidirectional link between stress, depression, and type 2 diabetes mellitus. Ann N Y Acad Sci. 2017;1391(1):20-34. doi:10.1111/nyas.13217
9. Centers for Disease Control and Prevention. Diabetes risk factors. https://www.cdc.gov. Published May 2023. Accessed July 5, 2025.
10. DeFronzo RA, Ferrannini E, Groop L, et al. Type 2 diabetes mellitus. Nat Rev Dis Primers. 2015;1:15019. doi:10.1038/nrdp.2015.19
11. American Diabetes Association. Standards of medical care in diabetes—2023 abridged for primary care providers. Clin Diabetes. 2023;41(1):4-31. doi:10.2337/cd23-as01
12. Centers for Disease Control and Prevention. National diabetes statistics report 2023. https://www.cdc.gov/diabetes. Published 2023. Accessed July 5, 2025.
13. Grundy SM, Cleeman JI, Daniels SR, et al. Diagnosis and management of the metabolic syndrome: an American Heart Association/National Heart, Lung, and Blood Institute Scientific Statement. *Circulation.* 2005;112(17):2735-2752. doi:10.1161/CIRCULATIONAHA.105.169404
14. Ford ES, Giles WH, Dietz WH. Prevalence of the metabolic syndrome among US adults: findings from the third National Health and Nutrition Examination Survey. *JAMA.* 2002;287(3):356-359. doi:10.1001/jama.287.3.356
15. Knowler WC, Barrett-Connor E, Fowler SE, et al. Reduction in the incidence of type 2 diabetes with lifestyle intervention or metformin. *N Engl J Med.* 2002;346(6):393-403. doi:10.1056/NEJMoa012512
16. Centers for Disease Control and Prevention. National Diabetes Statistics Report, 2022. Accessed July 5, 2025. https://www.cdc.gov/diabetes/data/statistics-report/index.html
17. Monteiro CA, Cannon G, Levy RB, et al. Ultra processed foods what they are and how to identify them. Public Health Nutr. 2019;22(5):936-941.
18. Srour B, Fezeu LK, Kesse Guyot E, et al. Ultra processed food intake and risk of type 2 diabetes. JAMA Intern Med. 2020;180(2):283-291.
19. Fardet A, Rock E. Ultra processed foods and food system sustainability. Adv Nutr. 2021;12(1):29-39.
20. Hu FB, Malik VS. Sugar sweetened beverages and risk of obesity and type 2 diabetes. JAMA. 2012;307(21):2260-2267.
21. Liu S, Willett WC, Stampfer MJ, et al. A prospective study of dietary glycemic load and diabetes risk. Am J Clin Nutr. 2000;71(6):1455-1461.
22. Johnson RJ, Segal MS, Sautin Y, et al. Potential role of fructose in metabolic syndrome. Am J Clin Nutr. 2007;86(4):899-906.

References

23. GBD 2016 Alcohol Collaborators. Alcohol use and disease burden. Lancet. 2018;392(10152):1015-1035.
24. Knott C, Bell S, Britton A. Alcohol consumption and diabetes risk. Diabetes Care. 2015;38(4):723-730.
25. Mozaffarian D, Katan MB, Ascherio A, et al. Trans fatty acids and cardiovascular disease. N Engl J Med. 2006;354(15):1601-1613.
26. Thompson FE, Subar AF. Dietary assessment methodology. J Nutr. 2014;144(7):1103-1110.
27. Chassaing B, Koren O, Goodrich JK, et al. Dietary emulsifiers impact gut microbiota. Nature. 2015;519(7541):92-96.
28. Suez J, Korem T, Zeevi D, et al. Artificial sweeteners induce glucose intolerance. Nature. 2014;514(7521):181-186.
29. Jianqin S, Leiming X, Lu X, et al. Effects of A1 vs A2 beta casein on inflammation. Nutr J. 2016;15:35.
30. Zhang X, Li Y, Del Gobbo LC, et al. Magnesium intake and diabetes risk. Diabetes Care. 2016;39(12):2116-2124.
31. Willi C, Bodenmann P, Ghali WA, et al. Active smoking and diabetes risk. JAMA. 2007;298(22):2654-2664.
32. Jackson CL, Hu FB. Inflammation and metabolic disease. Annu Rev Public Health. 2018;39:61-75.
33. Clore JN, Thurby-Hay L. Glucocorticoid-induced hyperglycemia. Endocr Pract. 2009;15(5):469-474.
34. Sattar N, Preiss D, Murray HM, et al. Statins and risk of incident diabetes. Lancet. 2010;375(9716):735-742.
35. Pan A, Sun Q, Okereke OI, et al. Antidepressant use and risk of type 2 diabetes. Diabetes Care. 2012;35(12):2540-2545.
36. Newcomer JW. Second-generation antipsychotics and metabolic effects. J Clin Psychiatry. 2005;66 Suppl 7:36-46.
37. Godsland IF. Insulin resistance and oral contraceptives. Am J Obstet Gynecol. 2005;192(6):1903-1909.
38. Hammerness PG, Wilens TE, Mick E, et al. Cardiovascular effects of stimulant treatment. J Clin Psychiatry. 2009;70(11):1491-1501.
39. Vincenti F, Friman S, Scheuermann E, et al. Results of an international randomized trial of tacrolimus. Am J Transplant. 2007;7(4):914-924.
40. Choueiri TK, Je Y, Sonpavde G, et al. Incidence and risk of hypertension with VEGF inhibitors. Lancet Oncol. 2010;11(6):543-552.
41. Huxley R, Lee CM, Barzi F, et al. Coffee, decaffeinated coffee, and tea consumption in relation to incident type 2 diabetes. Arch Intern Med. 2009;169(22):2053-2063.
42. Hosoda K, Wang MF, Liao ML, et al. Antihyperglycemic effect of oolong tea. Diabetes Care. 2003;26(6):1714-1718.
43. InterAct Consortium. Tea consumption and incidence of type 2 diabetes. Diabetologia. 2012;55(3):684-692.
44. Mozaffari-Khosravi H, Jalali-Khanabadi BA, Afkhami-Ardekani M, et al. The effects of sour tea on metabolic parameters. J Nutr Metab. 2014;2014:405917.
45. Kawano A, Nakamura H, Hata S, et al. Rooibos tea and glucose metabolism. Phytomedicine. 2009;16(6-7):437-443.
46. Khan A, Safdar M, Ali Khan MM, et al. Cinnamon improves glucose and lipids. Diabetes Care. 2003;26(12):3215-3218.
47. Mahluji S, Ostadrahimi A, Mobasseri M, et al. Effects of ginger on glycemic indices. Int J Food Sci Nutr. 2013;64(6):682-686.

References

48. Kato A, Minoshima Y, Yamamoto J, et al. Chamomile and glycemic control. J Agric Food Chem. 2008;56(17):8206-8211.
49. Weidner C, Wowro SJ, Rousseau M, et al. Lemon balm and metabolic effects. Phytomedicine. 2015;22(4):383-390.
50. Pittas AG, Lau J, Hu FB, Dawson-Hughes B. The role of vitamin D and calcium in type 2 diabetes. *J Clin Endocrinol Metab*. 2007;92(6):2017-2029.
51. Seida JC, Mitri J, Colmers IN, et al. Effect of vitamin D3 supplementation on improving glucose homeostasis and preventing diabetes. *Ann Intern Med*. 2014;161(3):195-204.
52. Guerrero-Romero F, Rodríguez-Morán M. Magnesium improves insulin sensitivity in type 2 diabetes. *Diabetes Care*. 2011;34(5):e65.
53. Simental-Mendía LE, Sahebkar A, Rodríguez-Morán M, Guerrero-Romero F. Effect of magnesium supplementation on glucose metabolism. *Diabetes Metab*. 2016;42(4):303-314.
54. Reinstatler L, Qi YP, Williamson RS, Garn JV, Oakley GP Jr. Association of biochemical B12 deficiency with metformin therapy. *Diabetes Care*. 2012;35(2):327-333.
55. Verhoef P, Stampfer MJ, Buring JE, Gaziano JM, Willett WC. Homocysteine metabolism and risk of cardiovascular disease. *Am J Clin Nutr*. 2002;75(5):908-915.
56. Forman JP, Rimm EB, Stampfer MJ, Curhan GC. Folate intake and risk of incident hypertension. *JAMA*. 2005;293(3):320-329.
57. Fernández-Real JM, López-Bermejo A, Ricart W. Cross-talk between iron metabolism and diabetes. *Diabetes*. 2002;51(8):2348-2354.
58. Jayawardena R, Ranasinghe P, Galappatthy P, Malkanthi R, Constantine G, Katulanda P. Effects of zinc supplementation on diabetes. *Diabetol Metab Syndr*. 2012;4:13.
59. Anderson RA, Cheng N, Bryden NA, et al. Chromium supplementation improves glucose tolerance. *Diabetes*. 1997;46(11):1786-1791.
60. Udovcic M, Pena RH, Patham B, Tabatabai L, Kansara A. Hypothyroidism and metabolic dysfunction. *Curr Opin Endocrinol Diabetes Obes*. 2017;24(5):377-386.
61. Whitworth JA, Williamson PM, Mangos G, Kelly JJ. Cardiovascular consequences of cortisol excess. *Endocr Rev*. 2005;26(2):115-138.
62. Hackett RA, Steptoe A. Psychosocial stress and metabolic risk. *Psychosom Med*. 2017;79(2):114-126.
63. Chrousos GP. Stress and disorders of the stress system. *Nat Rev Endocrinol*. 2009;5(7):374-381.
64. Harris MA, et al. Perceived stress and glucose metabolism. *Diabetes Care*. 2017;40(7):e87-e88.
65. Kyrou I, et al. Stress, insulin resistance, and obesity. *Nat Rev Endocrinol*. 2018;14(6):363-375.
66. Roberts AL, et al. PTSD and metabolic disease. *Am J Epidemiol*. 2015;182(5):397-406.
67. Mezuk B, et al. Depression and diabetes risk. *Diabetes Care*. 2008;31(12):2383-2390.
68. Ma X, et al. Breathing exercises and insulin sensitivity. *Front Psychol*. 2017;8:874.
69. Pascoe MC, et al. Stress reduction and metabolic outcomes. *Psychoneuroendocrinology*. 2017;80:63-74.
70. Creswell JD, et al. Mindfulness meditation and inflammation. *Psychoneuroendocrinology*. 2012;37(3):373-381.
71. Gore AC, Chappell VA, Fenton SE, et al. Endocrine-disrupting chemicals. *Endocr Rev*. 2015;36(6):E1-E150.
72. Heindel JJ, Blumberg B, Cave M, et al. Metabolism disrupting chemicals and diabetes. *Lancet Diabetes Endocrinol*. 2017;5(6):453-467.
73. Lang IA, Galloway TS, Scarlett A, et al. Association of urinary BPA with diabetes. *JAMA*. 2008;300(11):1303-1310.
74. Montgomery MP, Kamel F, Saldana TM, et al. Pesticide exposure and diabetes risk. *Am J Epidemiol*. 2008;168(11):1239-1246.

References

75. Kuo CC, Moon K, Thayer KA, Navas-Acien A. Arsenic exposure and diabetes. *Curr Diab Rep.* 2013;13(5):650-657.
76. Brook RD, Xu X, Bard RL, et al. Air pollution and insulin resistance. *Circulation.* 2013;127(6):684-694.
77. Trasande L, Attina TM, Blustein J. Chemical exposure and metabolic disease. *Health Aff.* 2013;32(5):967-975.
78. Cappuccio FP, D'Elia L, Strazzullo P, Miller MA. Quantity and quality of sleep and incidence of type 2 diabetes. *Diabetes Care.* 2010;33(2):414-420.
79. Spiegel K, Leproult R, Van Cauter E. Impact of sleep debt on metabolic function. *Lancet.* 1999;354(9188):1435-1439.
80. Leproult R, Van Cauter E. Role of sleep loss in metabolic disorders. *J Clin Endocrinol Metab.* 2010;95(9):4173-4181.
81. Spiegel K, Tasali E, Penev P, Van Cauter E. Sleep curtailment and appetite regulation. *Ann Intern Med.* 2004;141(11):846-850.
82. Reutrakul S, Van Cauter E. Sleep apnea and diabetes. *Diabetes Care.* 2018;41(4):683-695.
83. Gan Y, Yang C, Tong X, et al. Shift work and diabetes risk. *Occup Environ Med.* 2015;72(1):72-78.
84. Patterson RE, Sears DD. Metabolic effects of intermittent fasting. *Annu Rev Nutr.* 2017;37:371-393.
85. Sutton EF, Beyl R, Early KS, et al. Early time-restricted feeding improves insulin sensitivity. *Cell Metab.* 2018;27(6):1212-1221.
86. de Cabo R, Mattson MP. Effects of intermittent fasting on health and disease. *N Engl J Med.* 2019;381(26):2541-2551.
87. Anton SD, Moehl K, Donahoo WT, et al. Flipping the metabolic switch. *Obesity.* 2018;26(2):254-268.
88. Longo VD, Panda S. Fasting, circadian rhythms, and metabolic health. *Cell Metab.* 2016;23(6):1048-1059.
89. Colberg SR, Sigal RJ, Yardley JE, et al. Physical activity and diabetes. *Diabetes Care.* 2016;39(11):2065-2079.
90. Hawley JA, Lessard SJ. Exercise training-induced improvements in insulin action. *J Appl Physiol.* 2008;104(4):1074-1082.
91. Castaneda C, Layne JE, Munoz-Orians L, et al. Resistance training and glycemic control. *Diabetes Care.* 2002;25(12):2335-2341.
92. Umpierre D, Ribeiro PA, Kramer CK, et al. Physical activity advice and diabetes. *Diabetologia.* 2011;54(7):1634-1644.
93. DiPietro L, Gribok A, Stevens MS, Hamm LF, Rumpler W. Walking after meals and glucose control. *Diabetes Care.* 2013;36(10):3262-3268.
94. Hu FB, et al. Dietary patterns and risk of type 2 diabetes mellitus. *Am J Clin Nutr.* 2001;73(1):101–108.
95. Esposito K, et al. Dietary therapy in type 2 diabetes. *Diabetes Care.* 2014;37(6):1824–1833.
96. Barbagallo M, Dominguez LJ. Magnesium and type 2 diabetes. *World J Diabetes.* 2015;6(10):1152–1157.
97. Pittas AG, et al. Vitamin D and diabetes. *J Clin Endocrinol Metab.* 2010;95(12):5325–5333.
98. Clore JN, Thurby-Hay L. Glucocorticoid-induced hyperglycemia. *Endocr Pract.* 2009;15(5):469–474.
99. Joseph JJ, Golden SH. Cortisol dysregulation and diabetes. *Curr Diab Rep.* 2017;17(11):104.
100. Heraclides A, et al. Stress and risk of type 2 diabetes. *Psychosom Med.* 2009;71(7):733–739.
101. Mezuk B, et al. Depression and diabetes risk. *Diabetes Care.* 2008;31(12):2383–2390.
102. Spiegel K, et al. Sleep debt and insulin resistance. *Lancet.* 1999;354(9188):1435–1439.

References

103. Tasali E, et al. Sleep extension improves insulin sensitivity. *Diabetes Care*. 2014;37(3):707–713.

104. Umpierre D, et al. Physical activity and glycemic control. *JAMA*. 2011;305(17):1790–1799.

105. Heindel JJ, et al. Endocrine disruptors and diabetes. *Lancet Diabetes Endocrinol*. 2017;5(12):1007–1020.

106. Knowler WC, et al. Diabetes Prevention Program. *N Engl J Med*. 2002;346(6):393–403.

107. Pescatello LS, MacDonald HV, Lamberti L, Johnson BT. Exercise for hypertension: a prescription update integrating existing recommendations with emerging research. *Curr Hypertens Rep*. 2015;17(11):87. doi:10.1007/s11906-015-0600-y

108. Ross R, Janssen I, Dawson J, et al. Exercise-induced reduction in obesity and insulin resistance in women: a randomized controlled trial. *Obes Res*. 2000;8(3):171–181. doi:10.1038/oby.2000.20

109. Stevens VJ, Obarzanek E, Cook NR, et al. Long-term weight loss and changes in blood pressure: results of the Trials of Hypertension Prevention, phase II. *Ann Intern Med*. 2001;134(1):1–11. doi:10.7326/0003-4819-134-1-200101020-00007

110. Paluska SA, Schwenk TL. Physical activity and mental health: current concepts. *Sports Med*. 2000;29(3):167–180. doi:10.2165/00007256-200029030-00003

111. Cornelissen VA, Fagard RH. Effects of endurance training on blood pressure, blood pressure-regulating mechanisms, and cardiovascular risk factors. *Hypertension*. 2005;46(4):667–675. doi:10.1161/01.HYP.0000184225.05629.51

112. MacDonald HV, Johnson BT, Huedo-Medina TB, et al. Dynamic resistance training as stand-alone antihypertensive lifestyle therapy: a meta-analysis. *J Am Heart Assoc*. 2016;5(10):e003231. doi:10.1161/JAHA.116.003231

113. Inder JD, Carlson DJ, Dieberg G, McFarlane JR, Hess NC, Smart NA. Isometric exercise training for blood pressure management: a systematic review and meta-analysis. *Mayo Clin Proc*. 2016;91(3):327–334. doi:10.1016/j.mayocp.2015.10.030

114. Cui J, Yan JH, Yan LM, Pan L, Le JJ, Guo YZ. Effects of yoga in adults with type 2 diabetes mellitus: a meta-analysis. *J Diabetes Investig*. 2016;7(1):116–124. doi:10.1111/jdi.12394

REVERSING DIABETES
10 Natural Secrets to Reverse Diabetes Without Drugs

Dr. Joseph Jacobs, DPT, ACN

www.ingramcontent.com/pod-product-compliance
Lightning Source LLC
Chambersburg PA
CBHW052024030426
42335CB00026B/3267